BLACK AND MENOPAUSAL

of related interest

The Menopause Maze
The Complete Guide to Conventional,
Complementary and Self-Help Options
Dr Megan A. Arroll and Liz Efiong
Foreword by Dr John Moran
ISBN 978 1 84819 274 4
eISBN 978 0 85701 221 0

My Black Motherhood
Mental Health, Stigma, Racism and the System
Sandra Igwe
ISBN 978 1 83997 008 5
eISBN 978 1 83997 009 2

Overcoming Everyday Racism
Building Resilience and Wellbeing in the Face
of Discrimination and Microaggressions
Susan Cousins
ISBN 978 1 78592 850 5
eISBN 978 1 78592 851 2

BLACK AND MENOPAUSAL

Intimate Stories of Navigating the Change

Edited by Yansie Rolston & Yvonne Christie

Foreword by Iya Rev. DeShannon Barnes-Bowens, M.S.

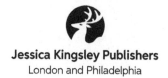

Jessica Kingsley Publishers
London and Philadelphia

First published in Great Britain in 2023 by Jessica Kingsley Publishers
An imprint of John Murray Press

2

Front cover image source: Halcian Pierre, Caribbean Neo Pop Artist
and illustrator at Art by Halcie.

Disclaimer: The information contained in this book is not intended to replace
the services of trained medical professionals or to be a substitute for medical
advice. The complementary therapy described in this book may not be suitable for
everyone to follow. You are advised to consult a doctor before embarking on any
complementary therapy programme and on any matters relating to your health,
and in particular on any matters that may require diagnosis or medical attention.

A CIP catalogue record for this title is available from the British Library and the
Library of Congress

ISBN 978 1 83997 379 6
eISBN 978 1 83997 380 2

Printed and bound by CPI Group (UK) Ltd, Croydon, CR0 4YY

Jessica Kingsley Publishers' policy is to use papers that are natural, renewable
and recyclable products and made from wood grown in sustainable forests.
The logging and manufacturing processes are expected to conform to the
environmental regulations of the country of origin.

Jessica Kingsley Publishers
Carmelite House
50 Victoria Embankment
London EC4Y 0DZ

www.jkp.com

John Murray Press
Part of Hodder & Stoughton Limited
An Hachette UK Company

This book is for all of us.

For all who have felt invisible while navigating the menopause space.

For the times we were overcome with shame and embarrassment,

and those times we were too scared to speak up.

For the way that our concerns were dismissed,
and our vulnerabilities ignored.

We are visible.

We validate ourselves and each other.

This is our voice.

These are our truths

and our stories deserve to be told.

Contents

Note from the Publisher

This book brings together a range of voices and experiences that for far too long have been missing from mainstream conversations about menopause. They highlight how experiences of menopause can differ depending on age, gender identity, cultural context and support from family, friends and healthcare professionals. The medical treatments and complementary therapies discussed in this book are personal choices that take into account each individual's unique circumstances, and we strongly advise readers to consult trained medical professionals before undertaking treatments or therapies mentioned in this book.

Foreword

Iya Rev. DeShannon Barnes-Bowens, M.S.

On March 8th, 2022, I was invited by one of the co-editors of this groundbreaking anthology, Dr Yansie Rolston, and two additional contributing authors, to speak on emotional wellbeing and menopause. This International Women's Day event was the first time I had been in community discussing the changes our Black bodies can and do go through as we enter and experience menopause. Listening to them courageously share their stories moved me to spontaneously speak about the relationship I had with my mother, and the ways in which she did not fit media-portrayed stereotypes of women who go through menopause.

Did my mother have hot flashes? Yes. I see images of her clearly in her early 50s asking whoever was driving to either open a car window or put on the air conditioner when no one else was hot. Did she suffer from brain fog, emotional irritability and chaotic mood swings? No. She was the same mother I always knew her to be.

While there was not as much focus on preparing me for

menopause as there was for beginning my menstrual cycle as a teenager, my mother told me in my young adulthood the basic facts about menopause as a natural part of a woman's life: 'You'll go through this when you get older and are about my age.' There was no fear or trepidation in her voice, similar to how she spoke to me about pregnancy and sex. I was reminded that our stories of ageing and going through natural life changes as women serve as medicine and teaching tools for generations to follow.

Black and Menopausal contains deeply personal experiences of vulnerability, courage, embarrassment, empowerment, pain, suffering, healing and liberation. This is the first time an anthology of this kind has been published. The collective voices of the authors are in alignment with a shift occurring throughout the African diaspora. Despite marginalization and invisibility, Black women and trans people all over the world are standing in their authenticity and taking charge of telling their own narratives with their varying sexual orientations and gender identities from different backgrounds and countries, and they invite us into intimate journeys about their bodies, reproductive health, sex and sexuality. As a psychotherapist who has specialized in working with clients around sexuality experiences and trauma, I have directly witnessed the positive transformative effect Black women and trans people experience when they have safe spaces and platforms to be seen, heard and taken seriously.

Historically, Black women's femmes and trans bodies, sexuality, health and wellness have been racialized, hypersexualized and/or ignored. The stories in this book exemplify inspiration and hope, even when grief, mourning and loss are present. In *The Way of Tenderness: Awakening through Race, Sexuality and Gender*, author Zenju Earthlyn Manuel writes: 'When we began to recognize a distinction between what we have been taught and what we directly experience as a true and authentic life, we begin to let go of erroneous images; we begin to see.'[1]

Co-editors Dr Yansie Rolston and Yvonne Christie have brought together a group of writers to help us correct our socialized visions of menopause, and to see ourselves and each other through a clear lens of honesty and truth. *Black and Menopausal* is a sacred offering to African and Caribbean people of the diaspora of all generations. May you see yourself and those you know in these testimonies. May the nourishing words in these pages help you realize it is your ancestral birthright to live a physically, emotionally, sexually, spiritually and mentally pleasurable life rooted in wellness as your body changes.

---

1   Manuel, Z. E. (2015) *The Way of Tenderness: Awakening through Race, Sexuality and Gender*. Somerville, MA: Wisdom, p.83.

Introduction

This Is Our Story
Yansie Rolston and Yvonne Christie

Historically Black people have never been afraid to tell their story.

Our culture is based on the passing down of oral traditions, and griots (pronounced 'gree-ohs') have always been an important part of our community and villages, as we share historical and cultural narratives. Storytellers are educators working tirelessly alongside leaders, helping to shape the politics of society, and it is storytellers and story keepers who help us to preserve our identity, to understand who we are in mind, body and soul, offering wisdom towards better health and wellness.

Discussions about the menopause are becoming widespread, and also very commercialized, and as we were seeing and hearing more about it in mainstream media, two of the key things that stuck with us as editors were: who was doing the talking, and did their stories resonate with us?

The long and short of it is that the space is dominated mainly by white professional women, and as people from the

African and Caribbean diaspora, we did not see ourselves in their narratives, and that was and still is very disconcerting because in the UK, where we both live, race is an important factor in the way that we experience life. It is almost as though Black women, femmes, trans and non-conforming, non-binary bodies are invisible, or that our stories not worth being told. But we are the very people who are known to be on the receiving end of racism, bias and prejudice in health and wellbeing services and in the workplace.

Those of us contributing to this book have not always been able to be open about our lived experience on several fronts, and as Black people many of us have been schooled to keep our business at home and among ourselves – a survival technique developed during slavery and colonialization that has been handed down through the generations. But we curated this book because it is important to give life to our own story and many other stories from different African and Caribbean diaspora, communities of diverse peoples, cultures and heritages, so that others can see themselves and know that there is more than one way to experience the menopause.

When we first started having discussions on the menopause way back in 2014, we were at two different stages in our own personal menopause journey and wanted to connect with others to better understand what we ourselves were going through. When did crying with laughter become weeing with laughter as tears would trickle down the legs? What could we do about the bald patch that was beginning to appear in our beautiful dreadlocs? How can we have that uncomfortable conversation with a partner about the tender breasts and sore vagina that was taking the pleasure out of lovemaking? So just as we, the co-editors, did, we hope that you, the reader, will also get a lot from the recollection of the various journeys in this book.

Onika Henry's chapter 'Menopause' educates in so many ways and is thought-provoking, especially against her imagination of growing older with joy. So many of us trundle along, not thinking about what happens to our bodies as we age, and her chapter sheds light on the benefits of awareness and resetting of the mindset. This chapter on ageing is juxtapositioned with Shaneka Lambert's 'Since I Was 12 Years Old' in which she recounts having to navigate premature menopause at a very young age and not having enough information and support, and the impact it has had on her desire to be a mother. The body is a temple, and we are reminded by Nicole Joseph-Chin in her chapter on 'Breast Comfort' that as we embrace menopause, our body changes and that the breast needs attention.

One of the major threads among many of the writers was the struggle with monthly menstruation/periods and the tide of emotions and feelings that this brought up. Palmela Witter, in 'My Black Panties', speaks of being a late developer in relation to periods, and its significance in the process of her identity as a Black woman. Many of the stories reflect moments of happiness at the prospect of no more pain, heavy bleeding and sexual interruptions that menstruating often brings, and that the prospect of the menopause was something that brought about a sense of freedom.

The complex interplay between wellbeing and slavery, colonialism, racism, bias and prejudice, and the inequalities and unevenness that come with that terrain, is shared by many. There are some uncomfortable experiences rooted in the 'medical gaslighting' of symptoms inappropriately down-played or dismissed. Yansie Rolston's 'I Will Take Up Time' sheds light on her experiences of prejudice and inequalities in trying to access quality healthcare and how it impacted her. Yvonne Witter's journey in 'Understanding My Limita-tions' also reveals some of that as she talks of her sexual and reproductive health challenges and the reasoning behind her mistrust of the healthcare system.

Austen Smith defiantly opens our eyes to the complex-ities of gender transitioning in 'Black, Trans and Menopausal', and how unprepared they were for the menopause. They also speak openly of coping on their own and how confused *everyone* was – including the medics.

Jacqueline Hinds, in 'Manifesting Wellness', shares in-sights into supporting herself and others as a menopausal Emotional Intelligence coach enduring racism and preju-dice in the workplace. As Black women, femmes, trans and non-conforming, non-binary people, we are often on the receiving end of negative microaggressive behaviours in the working environment, and not always given the empathy and support needed to cope with sexual and reproductive health challenges such as endometriosis, fibroids or perimeno-pause and menopause. This is despite research showing that women are more likely to have early menopause if they are Black, and 80 per cent more likely to have fibroid growths in the uterus by the age of 50. We are often conscious of negative judgements in the workplace, and this means we are reluctant to share our pain and health needs, especially knowing that we will not be treated with the courtesy we seek and with the confidentiality required. Sandra Wilson expands on this in her chapter on 'The Mask of Professionalism', reminding many of us who have been there, that NO, it isn't our imagination.

One observation from the various menopause group discussions we facilitated was that those from outside of the UK did not speak of the menopause as if it was some sort of disease that needed medicalizing, and so when Mbeke Waseme faced challenges in getting participants in Ghana to respond to her questionnaire, we reflected on that. Mbeke thinks that most of her potential participants didn't consider menopause a 'thing' but just part of a rite of passage. It was, however, very interesting to note in her interview with Mama K the many natural benefits derived from a regular Ghanaian lifestyle.

Even though menopause can sometimes cause debilitating symptoms, it is neither a disease nor a curse. However, the scaremongering that results from automatically following the word 'menopause' with 'suffering' and 'HRT' (hormone replacement therapy) is not helpful. Without science there would be no progress in so many areas of our lives – whether it be contraception, birthing, blood pressure and such like – and for some people HRT can be an absolute game-changer, but in reading the chapters embraced in this book, many of the contributors did not feel that HRT was their panacea despite many doctors and celebrities promoting it with such vigour. So where is the recognition that some cultures create and use complementary and herbal responses for their bodily changes based on Indigenous belief systems that have withstood being eroded and devalued by colonialism? There is a historical and cultural belief springing from our African ancestry that has been handed down through oral storytelling traditions that the Earth and feminine bodily functions are spiritually intertwined, and that lunar cycles influence menstrual, menopausal and sleep patterns. Maybe that is why many of the contributors displayed a desire to move away from chemical responses and seek complementary therapies. Our bodies are our temples, and we choose to treat them with reverence.

Asma-Esmeralda Abdallah-Portales shares her insights in 'Is HRT Really Necessary?' and speaks of the benefits she derived from using ginkgo, spearmint, red clover, milk thistle and herbs that mimic oestrogen levels in alleviating her moods. Pamela Windle reminds us in her chapter entitled 'The Return of the Pack' that even though some people struggle with debilitating hormonal symptoms as they transition into menopause, healing is possible. She, too, speaks of using alternatives to HRT. Based on the stories you are about to read, there is a sense that we intrinsically and knowledgeably know that taking HRT is not that simple.

How wonderful it would be if future generations could be more open, unafraid and knowledgeable about this time of their lives and have the ability to ask questions if they want to. Myrle Roach deftly reminds us in her piece 'The Invisible Cracks' that the generations before ours didn't tell us much, and that could be because they didn't know much themselves – they just cracked on with life. But the reality is that in critiquing the past for what our ancestors did not do well, we need to remember that our parents born in the 1920s and

1930s were much more circumspect and private about their lives – discussion on sex, for example, was a complete no-go area. Dr Leslie Anne Bishop, a practising gynaecologist, talks openly in 'Living My Best Life' about her personal experience negotiating the complications of sex during menopause, while Tashini Jones elaborates even further on this topic in 'My Fluctuating Libido', giving insights into her own sexual liberations and the fun she had along the way.

Menopause is not an illness, and even though sometimes it can be too hot to handle, for most people it is a natural occurrence, with a wide range of changes and symptoms. Yvonne Christie's 'More to This Than Sweats' speaks honestly about her vaginal prolapse, which was an unexpected change due to the menopause, but she also lets the reader know that she does not see it as her end-all. Instead, it is something she has adapted to and deals with in her own practical style.

The variety of experiences means that this book can be a catalyst for balanced menopause discussions, and a stepping stone in understanding the diversity of the journeys of pain, disappointment, growth, joy and laughter that have been our lived experiences.

We hope that sharing our stories will allow all ages to prepare, to learn and to resolve to ensure that their bodies are nurtured and loved. If you are lucky enough to get to that stage of your life naturally, the menopause can be cherished and relished, not run away from, and definitely not medicalized as walking towards a long dark road with dread of the 'final stage of life'. Remember that it is also quite possible to go through the menopause with very few symptoms.

Some of what has been written here is very uncomfortable,

but it is the strength of the collective, the community and the village that has comforted us as we speak of taboos and harness hope. Maybe it is the maturing that menopause brings that has given us more choice so that we are able to embrace happiness during the transitioning, and able to adapt and accept the changes. Having the ability to relax and welcome new terminology, learn new language and find solutions to our individual challenges has been possible as we came together in the intensity of community spirit to write this book.

It has been a great thing to turn up as our authentic selves on these pages and to offer some insight into who we are as Black women, femmes, trans and non-conforming, non-binary people in the African and Caribbean diaspora experiencing menopause. On these pages you will read our reflections of comfort, growth and resilience, see our over-laps, alignments and distinctions, and we hope that in bring-ing together these powerful testimonies, you, the reader, will leave with a better understanding of the Black experience of menopause.

1 Menopause

An Opportunity for Mindful Transition to Eldership
Onika Henry

The beginning

My menstrual cycle has always been consistent. I always
knew when it would come, plus or minus a day or two. And
so the first time it went missing, without any warning, plus
the accompanying brain fog and loss of memory, I panicked.
I visited the pharmacist and asked for medication to make
my period come. The period that has been intensely painful,
causing me much discomfort and inconvenience for more
than half my life – I wanted it back. If this was the beginning
of menopause, I. Wasn't. Ready.

I used to imagine ageing and growing old with satisfaction and joy. And so when I began to see the signs of the
so-called 'change of life', I instantly felt fear and sadness,
and this confused me. I was mentally and emotionally unprepared even though I knew that I was at the age and stage
when this was going to happen, and I wondered deeply at
my response. When did this image of ageing with satisfaction

and joy become fear, or, more importantly, why? What was different about me in my youth, compared to now, as I approached mid-life?

As I probed my mind and my heart, I realized that what had changed was my vision of my future self and the realities of the trajectory of my life at the moment. Ageing seemed a welcomed phase when I believed I would be married and have the perfect nuclear family, that all my debts would be paid off and I would be winding down my career and starting an adventure of travel, gardening and beach parties. I expected that ageing would bring an accumulation of resources, knowledge and accomplishments, and the expansion of my family through descendants – all the things that are deeply respected by the society I grew up in.

Instead, as a 'late bloomer', my career is now starting, I'm happily single and I'm only now beginning to show signs of being a 'successful adult'. A flood of messages stored in my memory came up about the horrors of going through menopause, and I instantly felt like I was getting old, which means I will be slowing down and less productive, and all of a sudden my goals didn't seemed like they would materialize.

I was struggling to recall the names of simple objects and people I had known all my life. Memory loss happened more frequently. I began to worry that it would happen during one of my workshops, while I was training or giving a speech. This was where the fear came from. If this brain fog surfaced during a presentation, it would be followed by anxiety and disrupt the quality of my work. My self-esteem would take a huge blow, and that was something I often battled with throughout my life. I wasn't prepared to let that happen. And so I needed to reframe my thinking about this stage of life. I needed to prepare my mind and body for this transition, and minimize any negative impact.

My process

And a woman spoke, saying, Tell us of Pain.

And he said:

Your pain is the breaking of the shell that encloses your understanding.

Even as the stone of the fruit must break, that its heart may stand in the sun, so must you know pain.

And could you keep your heart in wonder at the daily miracles of your life your pain would not seem less wondrous than your joy;

And you would accept the seasons of your heart, even as you have always accepted the seasons that pass over your fields.

And you would watch with serenity through the winters of your grief. (Kahlil Gibran)[1]

I spoke to no one of my sadness about coming to the end of my fertile years, a sadness that was palpable in spite of the fact that I had no intention of having any more children. I couldn't think of anyone I wanted to talk to about this – the consequence of being a bit of a semi-hermit and loner in a postcolonial society severed from the repository

---

1   Gibran, K. (1923) *The Prophet*. New York, NY: Alfred A. Knopf. Available at www.kahlilgibran.com/the-prophet.html, accessed on 26 August 2022.

of ancestral wisdom and lost in the individualism of a West-ernized worldview that denies us the support and container of community connections. I read.

In addition to the work of experts in the health and well-ness world of conventional and naturopathic medicating, I deliberately sought out books written from a non-white, non-Western perspective and books that shared about cul-tures with affirming and empowering messages about ageing. I read a lot and I cried some when my fear was more than my faith.

It was while reading a book on cultural anthropology that I came across information about the Ju/'hoansi of Botswana.[2] In this nation of people, elder caregiving is an important value and the responsibility of all adult children. The elders are independent and autonomous and are not considered a burden, even those who cannot care for themselves. Accord-ing to Joel Rosenberg, elders are associated with generative and life-giving activities in the community, are felt to have special powers, and may occupy strong leadership roles. The Ju/'hoansi elders are not afraid of pauperization or the anx-ieties associated with ageing in Western societies.

This was all I needed to set me on a course of committed self-care, improved nutrition and consistent exercise. I began to recognize that I didn't have to be stuck in the negative stereotype of the bitchy, moody, menopausal woman, who is un-sexy and whose mental health is temporarily offline during the transition. I especially want to be 'generative' and involved in 'life-giving activities'. What really stood out for

---

2   Rosenberg, J. C. (2003) *Nonviolent Communication: A Language of Life* (2nd edn). Encinitas, CA: PuddleDancer Press.

me, what I deeply connected with, was the belief that elders are 'felt to have special powers'. For me, this exactly matched my intention to become more involved in spiritual learning, training and activities – this is where I felt I could have 'special powers'.

Reframing the concept of menopause and ageing and buy-ing into this new view, or embodying it fully, did not happen overnight. It required a daily reminder that I was becoming fertile in other ways, that the end of my biological or earthly reproductive ability meant the beginning of fertility in other aspects of life. I reminded myself that a menstrual cycle, biologically, required a lot of energy to sustain, and that ending it was a way of prolonging life, and my hormones and creative energy were being redistributed. I reasoned that if I prepared for this, and kept my health reservoir full, then the transition would not be depleting and especially difficult.

A very helpful analogy for me is to think of the physical and emotional discomfort of perimenopause as labour pains. I see it as another development stage of life in which I am giving birth to a new and upgraded version of myself. My energy is now more for me and my new role as an elder. But I had to figure out who or what an elder is exactly, because while everyone grows old, it seems to me that not everyone becomes an elder.

Elders are not just repositories of knowledge and wisdom but are honoured by and have the respect of those in their family and community regardless of age. They are actively sought after because they are valued and do not have to demand submission or use inheritance as leverage or a bar-gaining chip.

For me, the most important step towards a better experience of menopause was adjusting my mindset. I focused on knowledge: knowing and understanding how the body works and how it changes; knowing where and how to get help, resources and information. I worked really hard on my beliefs. I practised accepting that this was a normal and natural part of life as a woman and not a loss of femininity or womanhood. I began to trust that there were ways to make the process better or less stressful. I practised new attitudes: I continued to be curious and open to new and different ways of thinking about womanhood and sexuality. I began to look for group support and started sharing and talking with others.

I learned that in addition to the hormonal shift that means an end to childbearing, women's bodies, and especially our nervous systems, are being, quite literally, rewired. In other words, our brains are changing. Our thoughts, ability to focus (that brain fog!) and the amount of nourishment going to the intuitive centres in the brain are all connected to and affected by this rewiring.

This literal rewiring of the brain means that a woman may begin to view life differently. I know that, for me, all significant relationships came under scrutiny. I began working more deliberately on healing any unfinished or unresolved issues from the past. As a late bloomer, I was still pursuing higher education and I began looking at courses and training in unconventional subjects, exploring and establishing an entirely new and exciting relationship with creativity and vocation. My energy became focused on working with my adult children as equals, rather than in a mainly supportive or parenting role. This 'new world view' also meant that I was very willing and okay with testing long-established relationships and accepting any disruption that came.

What was particularly important for me, as a sexologist, was to tap into the fact that pleasure is healing and that sex can be medicine. Sexual and erotic energy, after all, is generative energy; it is the energy of creation, and therefore a source I decided to access more regularly. According to Morten Kringelbach,[3] the things that bring us pleasure are actually very important sources of information. They motivate us for good reason. And understanding that reason, taking that reason into account, and harnessing and directing that reason can make us much more rational and effective people. In *The Pleasure Center: Trust Your Animal Instincts*, Kringelbach concludes that if we understand and accept how pleasure and desire arise in the complex interaction between the brain's activity and our own experiences, we can discover what helps us enjoy life, enabling us to make better decisions and, ultimately, lead happier lives.

I also know that the brain is the most important sex organ. Its capacity to house a vast reservoir of erotic imagery and thoughts, and its role as the storehouse for attitudes, beliefs and knowledge, means that it can always be accessed for sexual pleasure. To embody this new mindset meant taking specific steps to connect more deeply with my physical being. It meant integrating mind, body, heart and spirit in order to match my definition of an 'elder'.

At the risk of sounding morbid, I must also mention here

---

3   Kringelbach, M. L. (2009) *The Pleasure Center: Trust Your Animal Instincts*. New York, NY: Oxford University Press.

my new and emerging relationship with death. During the COVID-19 pandemic, I had to come to terms with the fact that death and grief were more common than ever before. But added to this is the fact that perimenopause means that I'm getting older, and I will start losing more friends and family. I've had to find a way to cope, to accept and find some semblance of peace amidst the chaos of the present and prepare for the future. And so I came up with two things:

1. The physics of death.
2. Faith in a Creator who designed the physics of death.

So my physics tells me that, after death, all our energy, every vibration, every measure of heat, every wave of every particle that is part of our human being-ness, is still a part of this universe, for energy is not destroyed but merely transformed from one form to another. And according to the law of the conservation of energy, not a bit of us is gone; we're just less contained and less orderly.

Ancient technologies for pleasure

As I write this now, I'm still in the early stages of my perimenopause transition. I've decided to take control of what I can, and one of my guiding principles is 'follow your pleasure'. This is not a declaration of my intention to engage in pleasure in an excessive, overly self-indulgent way, but as a way of being authentic and avoiding unnecessary self-sacrifice that is harmful and unhealthy for my wellbeing. My adapted version of a popular meme goes like this: if it doesn't bring me inspiration, income, peace or orgasms, I let it go.

What I call 'ancient technologies' are ancestral practices or tools such as genital steaming, jade eggs, using the expressive arts, herbal remedies, yoga, meditation, etc. I'm really curious about these and they inspire me to connect in natural ways with my self, my environment and the earth. These practices in their original cultural contexts require setting intentions, connecting to spirit (or whatever you consider to be a force outside of and bigger than yourself), developing a routine and some kind of self-discipline, and, of course, I get to discover new sensations, new pleasures and new joys. I explore breath work, movement, erotic touch, massage, working with ritual, meditation, and so much more, originating mainly from ancestral technologies, but all supported and informed by the neuroscience of brain and body.

I take charge of and responsibility for my moods, and I am mindful about my responses and reactions to life changes. When desire and joy don't emerge organically or as spontaneously as they used to, it means 'deciding' to choose them. I reach for the best I can in the moment, and I accept that sometimes that means finding less pain or less discomfort, when pleasure is not accessible. My ability to deliberately and mindfully slow down, to choose how I think and what I do next are among my most powerful allies in reinventing myself as my body and life circumstances change. My ability to get myself turned on by life is one of the most magical self-care tools and potent aphrodisiacs in the world.

I love rituals. They can facilitate the process of self-discovery and mastery over different elements of life and living. I love preparing for rituals, and the ones I enact or create usually involve my whole being: body, spirit, mind, emotions and soul. Rituals are critical, but to be honest I struggle with consistency because I get bored easily. So I've settled on changing rituals often, to keep things fresh and dynamic.

Important rituals for me and my ageing body include body gratitude practices and activities of proprioception and interoception. The wisdom and knowledge we get from our bodies is different from that which we receive from our cognitive brains. This wisdom and knowledge is stored in our bodies as narratives in images and sensations, about what is good for us and what isn't, about what is working and what's out of alignment, about what is safe and what is dangerous. When it comes to what's safe and what's dangerous, it's about more than just the wholeness and wellness of our bodies. In other words, it can mean a threat to more than what we think or believe, but also to what we care about, do, desire or crave for.

Some days my mood is just off and depression sets in without warning. In my training as a somatic sex educator, I learned that our feelings, emotions and moods (love, fear, excitement, relaxation, arousal, happiness, reverence and ecstasy) all have biochemical and physiological components that can be regulated with training and conscious practice over time. I have learned to slow down and take a sacred pause at these moments and reach into my toolbox of somatic exercises and activities. I remind myself that breath, movement and engaging my senses produce a discernible shift in consciousness and an equally distinct change in the way I feel. I have the power to move myself from a state of fear or anxiety into a state of calm, relaxed awareness just by working with and through my body, and my soul loves it. It's not always instant, but it is always helpful.

The last thing I want to share are my steps for staying in touch with myself and learning to tap into the wisdom that is within me and around me.

First, as I observe myself and my reactions and response, I am compassionate and gentle with myself, always. I acknowledge that my personal history, my tendencies and the communities I grew up in – religious, educational, work environment – all shaped and influenced me in ways I recognize and perhaps in ways I am yet to uncover. In this noticing, I look for what gives me pleasure in small and large ways: physical, emotional, mental and spiritual. I scan for my resources both internally and externally (family, friends, community, nature, etc.). I never forget to remember what I'm grateful for.

Second, I identify the problem and the issues. These are the ways that my shame, fear, guilt, self-judgement and other negative thoughts about myself and my body show up. Once again, I show myself compassion and kindness by gently releasing these negative and energy-draining entities with loving kindness, turning my focus to what is empowering, positive and pleasurable in the present moment.

Third, I choose thoughts and feelings that are pleasurable, joyful and encouraging, even if only minimally so. I then follow up with actions and practices that cultivate rich abiding experiences and sensations. As best I can, with whatever tangible and intangible resources I have, I create the conditions for the better vision of myself to flourish.

Fourth, I'm learning to be patient and let pleasure be my

guide constantly. Savouring the goodness and harvesting the healing in this process makes it easier and easier to access pleasure, which makes room for creative thinking and a passionate life.

2 Since I Was 12 Years Old

Shaneka Lambert

Shaneka's story is taken from an actual conversation she had with an older cousin. The conversation was recorded, and this is the actual transcript.

Shaneka, it'll be nice to know what you went through as a young person who has gone through menopause very prematurely, and all the implications and everything else that goes with that.

SL: Are there any specific questions that you're gonna ask?

One of the questions I was gonna ask was when you started it, and did the doctors confirm that that was what you were going through, did they talk to you about harvesting your eggs and anything else you want to tell me?

SL: Never, no, they didn't! They literally told me you should be fine from about a young age and I got to about 25ish, then they started to say that I might be able to have a baby, that's all they've been saying since the very beginning. Nothing about harvesting my eggs at all, and then last week they literally told me that I have no eggs and that my womb is really small, and my ovaries are too small so I might not be able to carry a baby at all, ever.

More recently they've changed my chances of having a child and have told me to consider looking for an egg and sperm donor.

So, if they had done it right at the beginning, they could have said let's grab her now and deal with that issue before it's too late. But nothing has changed. Since the age of nine, they knew from then because at that age they knew I had issues with my hormone levels.

Really?

SL: Yeah, the levels have not changed, they've been low since the age of nine, but only now they are telling me that I have premature menopause. So, it's been, like, how many years, 13/15 years.

That's ridiculous – could they not give you any hormones or anything to prevent it?

SL: They could have done that from the beginning because I might have had a few eggs then, but now I have literally, like, none. They could have taken them out before and tried to harvest them. They were literally giving me blood tests every single week, then their conclusion was that I was too fat, bearing in mind the levels didn't change.

Always, it's because you are fat, okay, but I lost weight now and nothing has changed. The level is still exactly the same, so what now? And now they literally just referred me to a specialist, so they are still trying to work with me, trying to get the right HRT and stuff like that. But literally nothing has changed since I was 12, apart from my weight.

See this is the kind of thing that needs to be out there, because anybody who is going through the same experience needs to know the foolishness that is happening. They need to know what's not being done. So that if they are out there experiencing the same thing, they can ask questions.

I had missing periods, from then it's been a rollercoaster ride and it's got worse and worse.

One thing I want you to do is to talk to any woman my age that's been through the menopause (gone through it early but I've finished now) – they will tell you how our bodies change and how your body kinda ages overnight and, of course, you are a young woman, so it is not normal for you to go through any of that shit at this age.

SL: The achy bones, the memory loss, the headaches, all that stupidness, the bad tempers. Oh yes, and the mood swings, oh my gosh! I literally struggle.

I can believe that, cause my kids told me, especially the boys, they used to hide because my menopause sorta clashed at the times when my daughter was on her period. So, there were constant battles in my house and the boys were so scared.

SL: Yeah, it's been really bad. I have been on the right HRT and my hormones are still crazy. I literally will be fine one minute and fighting or screaming the next, and Mom would be like, you need to stop this bla bla bla, and I'll be like, I can't control it, then I'll be all crying. It's awful. I get hot flushes and I sweat mostly during the night. I sometimes sleep on a towel to prevent my sweat from seeping through on to my sheets. It's so, so bad. So, all this since 12. My hormone levels have been low since then, so technically, they should have known from then.

Of course, they should have prescribed the right HRT before my body started to feel the effects of it, but no, they didn't, they just left me.

I think you are a bit of a champion, a champion of the cause. Have you ever put any stories out on the internet or anything like that about what you are going through?

SL: No, I've put one about fertility, not about menopause, but I was gonna do one about menopause in a video, but I haven't really had a chance to do it properly yet.

Just get it out there because it is very important.

SL: It is because I'm sure if there was more information available at the time it was happening, things might have been different, because when it started around nine, they thought that it would have come back again. They would say, 'It'll come back because she's still young.' But it never did come back, and I remember one time I was bleeding for about six months straight. It was thick blood and they said, 'Oh, it's fine, it's just the old blood catching up.' But it wasn't.

For six months?

SL: It was, like, this really heavy blood; Mom was, like, this is not normal. But they ignored what I was going through. One of the things they could have done is sit with me and talk me through the menopause. When I was in school, from Year 10 they used to give me a blood test every Tuesday, but my hormones were always low, it was always the same – nothing changed, and we're here now facing the same thing. They could have given me some other form of HRT or something but nothing, nothing!

Well, we know for a fact when it comes to Black people and seeking medical help, especially Black women in the field of gynaecology, we are at the bottom of the ladder.

I can see that.

SL: Maternal death rates among Black women are higher than any other group. The health carers just feel like, oh, Black women, they're strong so just leave them, they're fine. So I can quite understand why they just thought she is a young Black girl so they don't have to make an effort to do what they were supposed to have done. I bet you if I was middle-class white girl things would have been different. Now that I have the London doctors for me, I feel okay. I don't know if it's because there are more Black doctors why I'm feeling more comfortable.

You are better off at the London hospital because they do a lot of research, so they may view your case as research. You have choices here; you can select what hospital you go to.

39

SL: They don't speak to you like an individual. They treat me like a number. Whether they can do something or not, they get you to a point where you have to accept that this is it, this is how it's gonna be, and you don't get some kind of closure. But you need to know what's going on properly.

Yes, I want a decent outcome for you.

SL: Yes, same here, because I've always had unanswered questions and not really an explanation for anything apart from what I got from my own research. To me it's nature's cruel trick.

It's nothing anybody has done, nothing you've done that has caused it. But there are far better ways of fixing and working you through it than the treatment you have been getting.

SL: I just really want some form of HRT to help with the way I'm feeling and how the way my body is reacting to the menopause. It's all the symptoms that go with menopause.

The weight gain, because you know when have you worked so hard to lose all the weight, you don't want the weight to return. You don't want the hot flushing, the arthritis that kicks in because you don't have the right hormones in your body. You can develop arthritis, heart problems, and if you develop heart problems, you can't be on HRT, so they advise people to start HRT early.

SL: I didn't know that.

I just wanted to give you some awareness about that.

SL: They put me on the pill for a while; that didn't work for me at all. I was gaining weight, having headaches and all that. So, they took me off of that and left me with nothing, so I'm just waiting now. Who knows when I'll be able to be prescribed with the right medication? Every day is just so different because I don't know if I'm going be happy, if I'm going to be sad, if I'm going to be angry. I get it all.

Regardless, you must tolerate all those symptoms, which are very, very natural, but because of your age the one thing I would be more than anything else is angry. You can start having symptoms for a very long time, and it wasn't until I started doing work on menopause that I realized that there are 37 recognized symptoms of menopause.

SL: That is a lot, Wow, that's a lot of symptoms.

Because you're going through it prematurely, I wonder if it speeds up and the symptoms last less than, say, 10 years. I wonder what research has been done. I wonder what they can tell you about how long it lasts.

SL: Yeah, that's what I mean – they have not told me anything worthwhile. They just tell me the same thing – I'm gonna be hot and I'm gonna be angry. They don't tell you about anything else, some of the things are not pleasant, the issues like you are gonna be getting stiff, they should be telling you all that because you need to be prepared. They sent me for a bone density scan that was like a year or two ago, they said I got weak bones and stuff from menopause, but they also said I would be okay for now. I've now been told I must repeat the same test again.

Do you still go to gym? That's one of the best things you can do; women who are active during menopause don't seem to go through so much of the stiffness aches and pains; it's like they can almost keep it at bay because they are keeping their body really fit.

SL: I just feel like there's not enough information. I didn't know premature menopause existed until I was watching *Good Morning Britain* on the TV and there was a lady on there who I think was about 28 and she said that she had premature menopause. She explained what she was going through, and my mum was like – this sounds just like you. Then a few years later they said yeah, that's what you have. But I still did not know what it is.

They can't even say why I have got it. They just say that they don't know, so I don't know what's going on. They had said it's because I'm fat, but I've lost weight now. I told them that I've lost weight, but it is still the same. So if nothing has changed, what is it then? I feel like it was just a convenient excuse so they wouldn't have to look beyond that point. If they continued their research, I believe they would have prevented the loss of some of my eggs.

Did they refer you to a specialist?

SL: They referred me to a specialist when they wanted to

know what was going on with my HRT. They referred me in October and my appointment was February 2nd, so I had to wait a very long time even after losing weight, yet nothing much has changed. We're back to square one. That's when I started to get problems with my knees, my right knee hurts; when I walk, I can hear my knees grinding together. I've had hair loss right at the front, and at the sides by my temple is really, really thin hair. Towards the back I have a really thick patch and really thin patches at the front. How embarrassing! I had to cut my hair short to level it out and to make it seem less visible. Nobody tells you about this part of menopause. So that is where I'm at right now.

I'm amazed as a young person who is going through so much that you're not making it show that it is affecting you so much.

SL: All my friends around me are not having children at the moment so I'm feeling fine right now. But if all my friends and family were having children, I would be feeling some kind of way about things. I would love to have children in the future with the correct person, but that will come with complications because I can't have a child normally. That's going to take a while because the doctor gave me a 5 per cent chance of having successful IVF treatment, and even if that actually works, there's a chance of miscarriage because my womb is small, which could have an effect on the baby's growth. They never told me any of this when I was being diagnosed, and I think it could have also been slowed down if I was given the correct HRT.

They had told me 'you get dryness' so I went for a smear test and the nurse exclaimed – 'Oh my gosh, this is so small.' The test actually hurt a lot and was so uncomfortable.

Have you tried vaginal moisturizers, or vaginal dilators?

SL: What's that? Nobody ever told me about these. There's so much to digest, there is so much to take in, and because everyone is different, there are so many things that can possibly happen. I have been going through this since I was 12 years old – it's so much!!!

3 Breast Comfort

The Things We Might Miss (on the Journey)
Nicole Joseph-Chin

In the context of breasts, the definition of comfort can vary for many. But the need for self-awareness never goes out of fashion and should not be overstated.

Our prescriptive and contextual definition of self-awareness for women during menopause is closely aligned with the perception of breast confidence and the ease that women feel about any of their bodily changes. It took me a long time to discover that I had been on the path of becoming one of the most deliberately invested researchers and advocates of a totally unconventional form of empowerment.

Following my years in the corporate environment and my many years of anguish around my body positivity and the pop culture-inflicted perceptions about my breasts, there was a whole new significance for me when I began noticing just how many gaps there were inside of the whole discourse. After several years of self-discovery, numerous client consultations, a multiplicity of global speaking events and international fellowships, never-ending quests to engage in the most uncomfortable conversations and experiencing the many unforgiving moments of self-love that turned into desperation, I recognized that I had to become that person who would be the breast evangelist, the warrior and the champion of addressing the difficult subjects.

That was when I stumbled upon my courage and determination and realized that there was an important undertaking and that I was to be the Chief Evangelist, Chief Missionary and Unafraid Advocate for an anatomical expression that would change the ways we allowed our bodies to organically experience the menopausal journey. I had to break barriers, ignore the noise, get past the many challenges and fears, and find a way to defy all of the stereotypical stories of why it was improper to speak about breasts in public places.

It was not even the case of the elephant in the room, because there were bigger issues to address – issues that came in undefined types of 'pairs' – odd to even, larger to smaller, perky to pendulous, well to unwell – all larger than life and filled with many moments of angst, not only for myself but for women everywhere, in every single corner of the globe.

Beyond my own personal experience and journey, I had already seen thousands of women from all ethnicities, all walks of life, and especially those who thought that they were alone in this journey.

As with all matters that involve a sensitive subject, there are ways that will never be 'the right way', so there was only one solution – grabbing the bra by its straps and taking on the world in the challenge of making woman comfortable, girls confident, fathers and CEOs aware that breasts were not going anywhere, any time soon. The world was to be made aware of the value that empowering women with their bras could have on their bodies, their psyche and, most importantly, their presence.

Today, it is not without the efforts of evangelizing in the most compassionate and courageous ways that I get to encounter and solve issues that are still not considered urgent outside of the sphere of interventions in wellbeing, as part of an ageing discourse.

First, as a girl at nine years of age, whose body was rapidly developing and having no clue that puberty was here to stay for a while, and to say to me, this is only the beginning. To now, the present moments, of womanhood, where I am in my menopause, having to address my body confidence and, most importantly, my breasts and anatomical power as a woman, as a leader, as a teacher, and, most importantly, as an advocate. What did I miss along the journey?

Becoming fully engrossed in the subject for close to three decades has brought me to the point of freedom, and especially for creating that freedom for women, girls and societies, to wrap themselves in the sense of confidence knowing that the subject has come a long way, and we have, in many ways, been emancipated from the shackles of feeling conscious of our breasts and, by extension, our anatomy.

As a woman's body begins to change again in this 'third wave' of body development – outside of puberty, pregnancy (if experienced) and then menopause – it is vital to track the many changes that occur, and especially those relative to the breasts and the obviously visible anatomical differences therein.

Our personal references and track record of viewing

a transformation of this power have been seen in women whose confidence waned at the time they were entering menopause, discovering that there were changes but not aligning them to the menopausal experience.

Over many occasions of having consulted with women who may have made a deliberate point of having a consultation within our empowering spaces, it became more evident that from the time of their arrival and our interaction to the time when they would have departed, there was a great sense of self-awareness that made women well positioned and armed for battle – the battle of being assured that there was a plethora of solutions and that there was also a valuable and sustainably life-changing experience that would come out of our conversations, out of our interventions and out of our connection on this very personal matter.

What might we have missed along the journey? Breasts being one of the visible and defining anatomical facets, there is no doubt that it is relatively easy to detect changes both in density and in overall shape, and any proportionate changes to overall physical and physiological being. However, from the point of view of addressing the degrees of breast discomfort that women may face during the menopausal journey, we acknowledge that if you don't have a full appreciation or understanding of the potential of this correlation, it can be easily missed or even ignored. It may be regarded as simply a matter of being 'uncomfortable' and not fully adapting to the associated nuances and impact of being both a matter of discomfort and, in some cases, a hard subject to broach.

Having evaluated sample populations at diverse intervals over a number of years, this was adequate in allowing us to be inclusive in our findings around the value of overall comfort for the ageing woman.

Being able to cue in on the physiological adaptations and the many adjustments that a woman must make, due to her menopausal experience, may come as a surprise to some, especially since this anatomical discourse may sometimes seem irrelevant. It is, however, a necessary discussion to be had, and it is also an important facet of addressing the psychosocial aspects of the menopausal experience among women, its relationship with comfort and appearance, and adding a level of ease to the entire menopausal experience and the journey of ageing in general, through the lenses of breasts.

For many women, there is a concern around the changes in their breasts.

This situational discourse does not by any means reduce the validity of and necessity for medical or clinical research and histological findings or diagnoses, and is more aligned to the referencing of the experience of decades of dedicated and close engagement with women of diverse ages, varied stages of life, and especially a timeline dedicated to perimenopausal and menopausal women as part of their breast care and intimate apparel experience at my company, Ms Brafit.

Delving into a distinctive solutions-driven application for the overall achievement of confidence and comfort for women and engaging in deeper discussions, there remains a clear association with a woman's desire for comfort to become associated with a sense of guilt, shame or moving away from what may have previously been seen from the lenses of a traditional value system. Hence, the woman's comfort becomes remote to her natural anatomical changes associated with the menopausal journey.

It is obvious that there is a sought-out need for enhanced breast comfort for women, as their social self-agency increases with age. But what did we miss along the way to our comfort and ease of embracing our breast changes during the phases and changes aligned with the menopause?

Most evidence points to the acceptance of one's body changes – especially where women may not, at first, have recognized or been aware that changes in their breasts, once not aligned to a clinical diagnosis or medical condition not related to menopause, might, in most cases, become a manageable and solutions-oriented collection of interventions.

Here is a tale of three women – all breasts are not equal!

B is for 'bravery'

When a woman gets any diagnosis in her 50s, more than likely she might already be in an advanced phase of her career, she might have possibly been in an advanced stage of her role of parenting, if chosen, and she would definitely be in the throes of her mid-life.

At this crucial point of being challenged by any diagnosis, a woman like Brenda would reach out to someone she trusted to journey together with her. In this instance, Brenda bravely reached out for a helping hand to understand the dynamics of this new journey, while garnering the relevant support that goes with this aspect of a significant life change.

At this very defining moment in a woman's life, we had encountered a woman whom we could call nothing less than

Brenda the Brave, a mixture of bravery, confidence and the mettle to resist all negativity in a quest to heal, to embrace the loss of a vital part of her anatomy. We knew that this was an opportunity to be part of her healing journey, and, most of all, that we could encourage her not only to look great, but also to continue to revel in her feminine power, emerge with confidence into the spaces that she knew and had already occupied, with all of the dynamism and confidence of a woman who seemed to never have been affected by the fallout from the diagnosis. Today, *Brenda the Brave* continues to rely on our professional solutions and to embrace every step of her bodily transformation which requires the finesse that keeps things simple yet contained. A woman now in her late 60s, she appreciates her feminine power more than before, and stands in authority to encourage and connect us to other women who need to tap into their power.

C is for 'courageous'

With a heart of gold and lots of patience, this mid-40s woman saw her body make some radical changes during the lockdown in 2020 when she began working from home. As she consistently went about her chores and activities, it never occurred to her that it was not only from lack of movement and exercise, but also from hormonal and physiological changes associated with menopause. Having been diagnosed with an autoimmune disease years earlier, Cathy had chosen to use her many experiences to teach herself how to live, thrive and be happy. After many adaptations to become comfortable with her situation and health condition, *Cathy the Courageous* was now using a blend of tenacity, surrender and joy to show the world that working through all of the setbacks inside of a pandemic, a physiological disorder and an inevitable woman's health situation, all on the cusp of her 45th birthday, she was prepared to fight the greatest fight to resist complaining about her breasts, because she now understood that it had no real association with her status of working from home, but more to do with the time of her life.

Emerging with this sense of awareness, it was the best way for her to now attend to the next acts of self-care that had, at its core, allowed us to address her comfort and confidence in a systematic way and for her to find further compassion for herself in the future. She became more determined to engage in unconditional and unapologetic self-love, while allowing herself to evangelize on the virtues of grace as a superpower and as a pathway to bigger moments to behold. So, when her first diagnosis of mobility due to an autoimmune disease was compounded by her overall peace of mind, she chose to embrace an ageing body inside of a diagnosis that would lead to one of the best experiences of transformation and trust.

Today it's small wonder that this woman still uses a whimsical blend of humour and courage as her way of saying 'yes' to the adventures of body love with a cane and a zest for life.

J is for 'joyous'

Meeting Joni was one of the most empowering experiences to behold. Joni is a mother and grandmother whose breasts had been her biggest challenge all of her life. As a mother, she thought that she had lost the biggest opportunity of attaining larger breasts as a result of pregnancy and breastfeeding, as it didn't happen. So she turned to her surgeon for answers, and those answers were the catalysts to her new-found confidence – but only for a while. After years of wearing implants, she decided to explant to begin a personal journey of discovery. So, armed with her 'sagging menopausal breasts', as she referred to them, we embarked on a journey together to help her to embrace her joyous journey. Joni discovered that her joy was actually steeped in self-acceptance. Joni's new adaptation to joy became infectious, and has never left her since.

As Ms Brafit continues to develop, design and build interventions that support body acceptance, breast care and self-love, inside of a health justice framework, it is important to establish what this means to the amplification of health for women and girls, and especially for ageing populations and the future of the quality of life for girls and, by extension, women. Our dedicated focus on dignity is one of the catalysts to meaningful change in the discourse of the respect and responsibility that is required for administering inclusive, respectful and good health and wellbeing, unconditionally, continually and consistently.

Under the United Nations' Convention on the Elimination of All Forms of Discrimination Against Women (CEDAW), we have actualized the value of applying dignity and placing it at the core of all of our meaningful interventions, educational design and advocacy outreach partnerships.

For women, the continuous desire and quest for comfort

during menopause lies at the core of a plethora of situational needs and important conversations about their bodies. It is valuable to place context to their comfort, and to ensure that what we missed during the past decades and centuries of propelling breast health dialogues now becomes more inclusive, and allows perspectives around a blend of cultural sensitivity, clinical references, socioeconomic frameworks and legislative drafting to allow women to have dignity in their ageing progress and process.

4 My Black Panties

Palmela Witter

These are my memories of the onset of perimenopause while having and living with fibroids. It is one Black British woman's experience of reaching that pivotal age and time of life, and how fibroids, a hysterectomy and the perimenopause affected the quality of my life. You will get a sense of my journey to what I would call 'climbing towards the mountain top' – including the pain, the bleeding, the clots, the family and the sacrifices. Then, as I started to climb down the other side of the mountain, experiencing the good and bad 'tropical moments', the relief, the release and my feelings of attractiveness of being a woman again!

My womanhood has been 'supported' by 'black panties'!

Unlike many young women aged 11+ in the 1970s, I was a very late starter – my periods didn't begin until I was 16 years old, and for the most part my late teenage years were normal – that is, until after the birth of my son when I was 19 years old. My monthly periods became heavier, around 7–14 days, when I would bleed constantly, expelling lots of small blood clots, my stomach would be distended and I would be uncomfortable.

Fast-forward to 1988 and I am pregnant again, this time with twins. The gynae team examining me said that I had two fibroids the size of marbles and they would not grow because the babies needed the space in my womb. Well, that was a laugh because as the babies grew, so did the bloody fibroids! I looked like a bloated whale – carrying twin babies and two fibroids growing daily inside me, I looked like I was carrying triplets.

The fibroids

My stomach was constantly bloated, I had unbearable cramps and was so anaemic I was pale in colour – I looked 'grey'. I had no energy, constant tiredness plagued me all the time, and when it came to the weekend, all I did and wanted to do was sleep.

I did not initially question why this was happening to me, but when I eventually mentioned it to my GP, they gave me more pills! Now I come to think about it, my GP was a man – so what the f*** did he know about what I was going through? He would have learned the theory, but he would never have that lived experience; he would never know what it actually felt like. Gosh, on reflection, 'men' (opause) are trusted with so many intimate aspects of women's wellbeing and what their bodies are going through – I wonder how they know so much about what is best for us.

I must mention my clothing. Everything I owned was in the colour black – I always wore black trousers, black skirts, copious pairs of black tights and my favourite black panties. These were not your usual pair of panties. They were the traditional 'Marks & Sparks' (Marks & Spencer) full-bodied black panties. The pair of panties your mother would wear, the traditional full-fitting panties that covered your whole bottom! Today this type of underwear might be called the 'Bridget Jones knickers'. At no point could I wear any short frilly-type panties – no, they would not survive the constant use of period pads and being changed at least two or three times a day.

Wearing black panties was my security blanket because they helped to hide any 'bleeding' accidents I might have, as they would not show any leakage on my clothes. I ditched all the other panties I owned because it was easier to buy new black ones rather than spend time soaking them in a basin, then washing them with lots of antiseptic!

So, when my periods started, what a bloody shock for me it was – I bled like a trouper. My mum had to buy me large quantities of sanitary towels, which I sometimes used with the elastic belt – that one you put around the waist with the two clips that would hang down and clip to the sanitary towel. It was either that or suffer the further indignity of having to wear two pairs of panties to hold the pads in place for extra protection. Boy, young people would die of shame if they had to wear something like that today!

In writing this chapter, I am reminded by one of my twin daughters that I used to 'walk funny, like something was stuck up my bum'. I asked her to elaborate, and she said that she knew I was in pain, but she saw me walking in a weird way to compensate for the pain I was going through.

That was because of the suffering I was going through with the fibroids and the impact this was having on my life. What quality of life did I have? I was in constant pain, suffering cramping, bloating and excessive bleeding, and it was not only my physical health that was affected, but also my family and work. It was at this time that I had to consider whether to have a hysterectomy.

The decision to do this was in some respects an easy one, but the one issue that was playing on my mind was that of being 'cut'. I had never had any medical procedure before – not even when having my children was I cut (vaginally or via a C-section), and so I was very scared indeed.

After having the full hysterectomy, where I kept my ovaries but my womb was removed (I am trying to fully reflect on how I felt at that time – I call this my grieving time), I was ever so glad that the 'thing' that had caused me years of pain, discomfort and incapacity was finally removed from my body – something like cutting the umbilical cord – it was finally gone!

When people talk about grieving, it mostly relates to the death of a loved one, but at no point in the run-up, during and following my hysterectomy did I ever articulate that I had actually lost a part of my body, even though it was an internal organ, and as I reflect now, was I offered any counselling? I do not really remember if I went anywhere, and if I did, I am particularly sure there was no culturally specific counselling available – that was unheard of.

Reflecting on my womanhood, I now consider what, if any, support agencies were available. I ask this question because when I was in my early 20s and experiencing heavy bleeding and clots, there were a few Black woman organizations that specifically provided support, advice and information on fibroids. I went to these organizations for support and advice, but in my experience, I found them to be mainly focused on steering Black women 'away' from having hysterectomies because of suspicions about the high numbers being offered surgery as a first resort.

I also needed 'help and support' in understanding what was really happening to my body and the possibility of having such an invasive medical procedure. I really didn't have anyone to talk to about what was happening to me internally, and what it all meant for me being a Black woman! None of my friends were experiencing or had experienced what I was going through, so I didn't feel that I could open up to them.

After the surgery, I then had to adjust to how my body now felt and what it looked like with a long scar on my stomach. It took me a really long time to even look at my body in the mirror because I was scared it would look deformed. The postoperative recovery was equally difficult, and that ultimately impacted on the healing process. It took over a year before I could return to work.

What helped with the recovery and healing was the photograph I had that was taken of my womb which showed the number of fibroids attached to it. Grotesque, some might say, and in some ways having the picture was like still having the fibroids, but it helped me. It was over a year later that I was able to finally exorcize the 'loss' of my womb by throwing away that picture. Acceptance finally came.

The perimenopause and menopause

Once I had the hysterectomy, I then went into the perimeno-pause stage. But what I experienced at this stage of my life did not really faze me. I do not recall if I was ever informed of what was to come, and if anyone was to ask why I was not fazed by the symptoms of perimenopause, it's because I had spent the previous 10–15 years of my life living with constant bleeding, bloating, discomfort, cramping – this was my norm – and I knew nothing else or anything different.

I considered the onset of perimenopause and the 'tropi-cal moments' – the symptoms of hot flushes, night sweats, mood swings – all blessings to me. I embraced those symp-toms because they were a welcome relief from what I had previously experienced over the past 10–15 years. So, when I hear of other Black women who say they suffered because of these symptoms, it was not my experience. I am not saying that some don't suffer – it is just that I did not.

I do remember the GP prescribing me hormone replace-ment therapy – namely, HRT tablets – to combat the 'tropi-cal moments' I was experiencing, but they made me very irritable and bloated, and I had water retention problems and suffered 'cankle ankles'. It was during this time that my ex-mother-in-law died, which was a very stressful time, and I stopped taking the tablets. A year after my hysterec-tomy, the symptoms of the 'tropical moments' did start to become unbearable. Did I have sweaty moments? I really cannot remember, but I do remember the night sweats in the bed, the on–off syndrome where one moment I was hot and then the next I was cold, and despite the weather, the window was always cracked open so I could feel a breeze. Surprisingly, these symptoms crept up on me – I didn't see them coming, and it took me some time to realize that what I was experiencing was the menopause. That realization sent me into another phase of thinking about me as a woman – my womanhood was being challenged.

First, I had spent the 20-odd years bleeding like a trooper. Second, I then made the life-changing decision to 'get rid' of the thing that was causing the bleeding – the fibroids. Third, having these symptoms of 'tropical moments' meant to me that I was finally coming to the end of what it meant to be a woman. All these stages of womanhood meant it took me some time to process the emotions, how I felt about them and what they meant to me.

Sexy black panties

I have asked myself, how can my story influence other Black women – the next generation of young Black women as they approach that phase of womanhood?

Well, I would hope that sharing my lived experience of having surgically induced menopause and having lived with fibroids during the 1980s will at least get them talking and sharing their own experiences. That it will take away some of the mystery. Yes, thankfully now medical advancements in treating fibroids prevents the majority of women from needing invasive hysterectomies, but some will still have early menopause.

What I experienced during my 20s and 30s I mostly ex-perienced alone, or at least it felt as though I was alone.

Yes, my mother was around, but I did not really confide in her, I didn't go into any great detail as to what I was going through, but she knew it, she saw it, and we did not really speak about it. That is despite my mother being a nurse and a midwife from Guyana who had also suffered from fibroids. The difference was that she did not experience the same level of discomfort and pain, and, dare I say it, she pushed through what she experienced and her fibroids had shrunk in size as she reached the age of 50. Apparently, fibroids are known to shrink after menopause.

This 'black panties' chapter is really about my experience of having to live nearly every day for around 10–15 years in full-bodied black panties that did not make me feel like a sexy woman. Those panties were plain and boring, and definitely did not make me feel attractive. How could I feel attractive when I was in such discomfort?

Now, 20 years after having my hysterectomy, I want Black women to know that they are not alone. Today there are many more support mechanisms available, we have the internet, and the young Black women of today are far more clued up on how the body works, when things are going right and when they are not, and when and where to reach out for help, advice and support.

I am now a far more confident Black woman, having exorcized the grief of getting rid of the fibroids that were part of my body.

I'm now in my 60s, and I do still wear my black panties, but these are more the lingerie style – sexy, frilly, lacy – and I love how I look in them, and so does he!

5 I Will Take Up Time

Yansie Rolston

I cannot begin to tell you how worried I was and how many hours I spent telling myself that no matter what, I couldn't be a burden on my family! Yet I didn't know what to do as it was obvious that my memory was fading, and confusion was running full speed ahead to take its place. 'Theatre tickets for 7.30pm on the 17th June' was what came out of my mouth, but my brain meant 'Theatre tickets for 6.30pm on the 17th April' – one hour, two months makes a huge difference in the diary.

The fear that dementia was galloping towards me was real; it just would not shift from my mind. Then I found my car keys in the fridge, and that was the 'straw that broke the camel's back'. The key rack is not anywhere near the fridge – they are at opposite ends of the room, and as a fast car enthusiast, I know that engines sometimes need cooling down, not keys. The moment I opened the fridge and saw the keys next to the butter, I felt I was being robbed of my sanity, so, in between the sobs, sweating palms and heart palpitations, I phoned the GP surgery for an appointment. That itself is an anxiety-inducing experience, because if there ever was an award for the rudest receptionist, the one at my GP surgery will be a serious contender, and, true to form, on that day she didn't disappoint.

In her usual dismissive tone that makes me feel like I am merely an annoyance taking up her precious time, she berated me for not calling at 8am. 'Call back tomorrow,' she said! I remember spending most of that night counting down the hours, and at 7.55am, with shaking hands, I dialled the GP surgery. How can I be number 9 in the queue when it's only just gone 8 o'clock? I shout at the awful background music. After holding on for what seems like an eternity, Ms Rude Receptionist eventually answers and my heart skips a beat. I can hear my own voice mumble something about calling yesterday and not getting an appointment. She responds in her usual 'Why are you bothering me?' tone. 'Well, you need to call back tomorrow. We have no more appointments for today.' I hang up and sob until the tears form a snake-like pattern down the front of my T-shirt.

I go through another distressing day and a long night, and bright and early the next morning I join the back of a queue outside the GP surgery, edging forward slowly as people get attended to. I'm pleased with myself because it seems that physically turning up has worked. I get an appointment for later that day and return 10 minutes before the scheduled time. 'What brings you here?' the GP asks. 'I'm losing my mind,' I respond, and proceed to rattle off the instances when forgetfulness reigned. He fires off a few more questions and surmises, 'It's the menopause, but because you've had cancer, you can't have HRT.' The consultation then becomes an update on my cancer recovery, with no further mention of the menopause. The sheer relief of hearing that I don't have dementia is overwhelming, and I leave on a high, grinning from ear to ear. It's only later that evening it dawns on me that I have no clue about the menopause. I begin to worry, which makes the anxiety resurface.

My gynae health matters

A genetic disorder means that I have a long history of navigating the healthcare system, and have built up my resilience by not taking medical advice at face value but always deciding to question, read, research and advocate. When necessary, I use my pen and keyboard as a weapon against failings in the system by highlighting them and raising awareness.

I don't like being treated like an inconvenience and once challenged a nurse who furrowed her brow as I was writhing with excruciating period pains and haemorrhaging through two maternity pads as she dismissed my symptoms as minor, at the same time raising her voice so that others could hear, to let me know that the GP had 'a lot of patients to see' and that I should go home and have ginger tea. Luckily, I stubbornly insisted on seeing the doctor and ended up having surgery and a blood transfusion! I also stood my ground with a Middle Eastern doctor who, on seeing me writhing in agony, said that I should be able to cope with the pain because 'where he comes from, women are strong and don't make a fuss'. I did have to remind him that his condescending tone, ignorance and medical sexism was not acceptable, and then asked to be seen by another doctor who took the time to listen to me. Within half an hour, I was being rushed into the operating theatre because of an ectopic pregnancy. These are just two examples of when I refused to put up with medical gaslighting, the minimizing of my crippling symptoms, and being made to feel small and insignificant.

Representation matters – race, gender, ability, class, education, colour, sexuality, age, etc. matter – but they can be used to do a disservice. Who feels it knows it!

I don't see me

When the euphoria of knowing that I wasn't descending into a spiral of early dementia subsided, anxiety quickly rushed in. Confirmation from the GP that I was experiencing menopause symptoms gave an explanation for the persistent fluctuations in my body temperature, but my mind took a leap into the future and landed in a place of fear and uncertainty, a place where I suddenly felt great discomfort in my body, conjuring up images of decrepitude because then my only understanding of menopause was that it was a gendered, age-related illness spoken about in hushed tones, and overhearing gossip about a person who disgraced herself by having a 'menopause baby', someone whose husband left her because she could no longer have sex, or about the co-worker who wore wigs to cover up menopause hair loss. I wanted to detach from the truth of what I thought was happening to me based on my limited knowledge, but curiously I also wanted to know what lay ahead. I consulted 'Dr Google' and lost myself in it for hours. I scrolled and scrolled, delving into the research, the newspaper stories and blogs – basically, I was absorbing any information I could find, but then it dawned on me that the information was invariably accompanied by images of white bodies that didn't represent me. That really caused me to question where the Black lived experiences are, the data on Black bodies – not even the tasteless sexist menopause jokes or cartoons featured Black skin!

My next source of information was to check the then popular online bookstore that has gone on to become a US$1401 billion business as of 2022, and that was no different, so off to YouTube menopause posts I went, and surprise, surprise, Black faces were not visible there either. Where my people at? Where are those images that look like me, those stories that I can relate to, those who have felt the pinch of the structural and institutional racism and discrimination? I don't see me!

Suffocating under the blanket of anxiety about my impending descent into what I thought was the disease of menopause, I reached out to some sister friends. I felt the need for connection and a solid support system of kinfolk. I remember vividly that the first one I confided in about my experience at the GP's and the anxiety I was having strongly advocated that I demand the GP put me on HRT – she said it made her feel whole again – but in the moment, I heard my own truth, and it was that I felt whole despite the anxiety I was experiencing, and, in all honesty, she, too, was very forgetful and constantly complaining about feeling overwhelmed, so I couldn't discern from what I could see outwardly the difference HRT would make for me. What I really wanted was someone to tell me that I'd be okay, and knowing what I know now, what would have helped me was hearing that not everyone has the same symptoms and that menopause is not some terrible disease out to prematurely curtail my life.

I needed reassurance from those with Black bodies, especially those with lived experience of the significant health inequalities in the UK. I needed to know that it is possible to have a positive menopause experience and that it is not always about a devalued, diminished identity trait. But what I got were statements embroiled in shame and stigma, some truly unhelpful gender biases, and suggestions of products and potions ranging from antidepressants to eating raw garlic.

Belonging

It is that need for reassurance that led me to reach out to friends, friends of friends, relatives, and, in some instances, total strangers on the internet, and I also wondered about visiting places where they are majority Black populations to root my experience in cultural contexts. The starkest cultural difference between the conversations in the UK and those I had in the Gambia, Côte d'Ivoire, Senegal, Cape Verde and some of the Caribbean islands was the way that they normalized menopause and considered it to be a rite of passage into eldership (not ignoring the fact that it can sometimes happen prematurely). I remembered being in awe listening to how eldership is centred around maturity, dignity and wisdom – 'The young bird does not crow until it hears the old ones' (a South African proverb) – and how the use of oral narratives, songs and poetry are used to pass on knowledge and give guidance to members of the community so that as they pass through life, things don't really come as a surprise.

Even though they saw me as different – they found my accent unusual and my hair colour intriguing – the magnetism between the people and me, and the love and patience they showed, mattered. I took up their time and they indulged me with story after story of their lives, of how they transition into eldership and the importance of ancestors, and I felt belonging. I watched, listened, learned and evolved – the more I heard the stories, the more I understood myself, and once I saw from their perspective the correlation between identity, culture and interpretation of the menopause, I anchored a sense of healing and empowerment. 'It takes a village to raise a child' is an assumed African proverb, and I became their child, and was more intentional and mindful in who I am.

Menopause was then no longer the life-limiting disease that my ignorance and lack of knowledge led me to believe it was. I found solace and solidarity, shifted my perspective and no longer focused on the ever-increasing list of symptoms (varying from 34 to 42) that we get told are synonymous with menopause. UK society's expectations or stereotypes of what menopause should look like were no longer at the forefront of my mind – you know the ones I mean? The unhelpful media messages and adverts that purport to halt menopause symptoms of sagging skin, wrinkles, age spots and crow's feet. I no longer let them hurt my self-esteem. Instead, I decided to use what I learned on my travels – to pay attention to my overall health and wellbeing, my mind, body and soul, and to use wisdom, curiosity and dignity when engaging with others. Truth be told, I did wonder how that would play out for me as a Black person in a society where youthfulness and young bodies are idolized, one where there is a growing infatuation with looking young and false perceptions of perfection. The saying 'Good black don't crack' or 'Black jeans/genes don't fade' is a source of pride for many as it exemplifies the phenomenon that among Black people the effects of ageing tend not to be as obvious as other ethnicities. But because I am a person full of contradictions, I embraced eldership and the lessons from my travels while also indulging in some stereotypes – I thank my parents for the youthful genes.

Living in my authenticity

I can assure you that it took some doing to reevaluate and reconstruct my way of being, and I still don't have all the solutions. I take the journey as it comes. I am a creative person, and leaning into my artistry means that part of me living in my authenticity is using my body as a canvas for self-expression. So, aligning my action with my intentions, I took the clippers and birthed a new Mohawk-type hairstyle, saying goodbye to long locs and the thinning, receding hairline that I had been covering up. After that, and on the insistence of the elders in Benin, my head was clean-shaven, and the regrowth is now without the patches and far-back hairline.

To manage brittle nails, I keep them short but painted in bright orange colours using the concept of chromotherapy, which is a healing modality that uses colour and light. The warm orange colour is said to be connected to creative, sensual and emotional energy, and my brightly coloured orange nails give me joy. Increased washing and sanitizing during the height of the COVID-19 pandemic forced me to moisturize my hands more often than I normally would, because lovely nails and dry flaky hands just don't go well together, and I am sure my hands are happy for the attention.

My wardrobe carries an array of loose-fitting statement layers – light cotton vests, jackets and blazers in various colours are a staple in helping to regulate my body temperature, and I accompany them with large belts to give the illusion of a cinched waist. Vaginal atrophy was the bane of my life, and the skin on my vulva would be painfully sore and red raw, so no more nylon or Lycra dental floss-type underwear for me; instead, it's cotton boy shorts, and during the time when a cough, sneeze or laugh was accompanied by a urine leak, I resorted to disposable pull-up underwear. Thankfully, that is now in the past.

Prebiotic inulin chicory extract fibre is part of my daily regime to minimize the chronic IBS due to a genetic disorder, but it also aids digestion, improving the nutritional value of certain food products, and minimizes the risk of me having diabetes. Even though I don't normally like sweets and couldn't stand the taste of chocolate (don't judge me – I know that I am in the minority with that one), once the postmenopause journey started, I began craving two squares of chocolate daily, and if I succumbed to the temptation, I inevitably got what can only be described as electric shocks running through my body.

I wear waist beads that were tied on my body on one of my trips on the African continent. They have a deep, cultural, rite-of-passage significance, and are viewed as a symbol of sensuality, femininity and spiritual wellbeing. Because they are never removed, I immediately notice changes in my shape and weight in the mid-section, so I can easily identify any foods that cause me to bloat, and the feeling of them rubbing against my skin is therapeutic, and I have to say that I like what I see in the mirror – they look sexy.

Incorporating botanicals and herbs as well as performing cleansing rituals such as smudging, burning incense, scented candles, wax melts and aromatherapy diffusers definitely help with my stress levels and insomnia, and my home is often an explosion of fragrances, much like you get when you walk through the duty-free at Heathrow Airport, and that reminds me of happy holidays. I find room humidifiers incredibly helpful because the additional moisture in the air makes my breathing easier, and makes a difference when the cold winter air and dry summer air evaporate the moisture on my skin and hair and replace it with grey-ash and rough sandpaper-textured lips.

Although there is no real scientific evidence that supports crystal healing, and some say it's the placebo effect, I have a collection, and just in case, I have rubies to restore vitality and energy and promote sexuality and sensuality, sapphire to attract happiness and enhance positive moods, bloodstone to promote selflessness, creativity and ideas, and moonstone to soothe stress and support positive thinking. Maybe it's simply the power of suggestion, but that's good enough for me.

As I put one foot in front of the other on this journey, I continue to find comfort, community, liberation and ac- ceptance through reconnecting with the traditions of my enslaved ancestors, and even though much is still misunderstood of these traditional practices in the Western world, it helps me to understand the discrimination, struggles and resistance they fought against to find peace, happiness and joy, and it is joy that I am after.

Reclaiming power

My menopause journey has been a rollercoaster, amplifying the fragility of life but conversely enabling me to see and understand myself within a much larger context. I have been transparent and shared with others, and that has created connections that have inspired and empowered me. I have been brave and vulnerable, showing up in raw form, and trusting the process of letting others in on some of my deeper secrets. I have done that even when being triggered but holding fast to the belief in the love and support of those in the space. I have been open to questioning and learning – asking hard questions, listening intently and deeply to the responses, paying attention to what is not being said and taking on board the knowledge and information shared. I have challenged the healthcare system, refusing to be treated with scant courtesies or blatantly ignored, and advocated on behalf of others to collectively illuminate our life's journeys. I believe that I am worthy and that I am good enough.

I finish by saying that pouring into myself has been a challenge. Maintaining balance continues to be a struggle, so I am being gentle with myself, practising self-care and self-comfort as I settle into postmenopause eldership. I face this wonderfully beautiful phase of my life with its ups and downs and embrace new experiences with gratitude. If appropriate, I will consciously take up space and time, stand my ground, reclaim my power, and I will do so with joy.

6 Understanding My Limitations

Yvonne Witter

My experience of the menopause was quite stark because my periods stopped in my late 30s. I was enjoying my life, work was satisfying and stimulating, and I had a decent home. I had been divorced from my first husband and had custody of our child, but he and I co-parented and were friends. What precipitated our parting is that I had foolishly expected a rekindled relationship with a childhood sweetheart to morph into something solid like marriage, but it never did, even though the idea of me having his child seemed to have been a great ambition of his. To this day, I am so pleased that I never had a child with him because it took me a few years to settle my heartbreak after that crushing disappointment.

They say menopause can be induced by shock, and maybe that was it. Uprooting for a love that did exist, but not in the way that I thought it existed. It is as if this man had me on a leash for decades, renting space in my head and heart. I had to wonder if he had been to see an obeah man,[1] such was my deep-felt commitment to this childhood romance that spawned when I went to Jamaica from London at 10 years old. My adoptive parents had decided that England was not the land of milk and honey after all and therefore sold up and returned to glorious sunshine, with me in tow. It was a move that was the catalyst for 90 per cent of my family returning to Jamaica in the late 1960s and early 1970s.

Word got out regarding the numerous opportunities to run a small business with capital that a healthy exchange rate provided. Restaurants, grocery shops, hairdressers, night clubs and bars and even an imported Mr Whippy ice cream van – yes, my family did all of that with the money accrued from house sales in England rather than toil in the cold, grey, hostile 'motherland'.

At age 13, my then boyfriend and I were gazing at each other across the Anglican church pews, him in his altar boy red-and-white robes, and me in my Sunday best. I don't recall what we talked about for hours on end as children, but I just know we spent a lot of time on his veranda after church with his other siblings talking. We walked around a lot too. That east coastline was beautiful, and staring out at the glistening blue waters was our favourite pastime.

I used to get the occasional parcel of clothes and shoes from England, so my gear was the envy of others. I really cherish the 10 years I spent in Jamaica, and had I not been shipped back to England in my late teens, I might never have

---

1   An obeah man is one who uses certain spirits or supernatural agents to work harm to the living, or calls them off from such mischief. See www.historyworkshop.org.uk/the-racist-history-of-jamaicas-obeah-laws

left voluntarily. The only thing I missed about London was the fish'n'chips, Crunchie, Topic and Lion Bars – if you know, you know. That was replaced by daily freshly cooked and tasty Caribbean food, and mango, June plum and Otaheite apple, which, back then, were my favourites. We are what we eat, they say, so had I continued that trajectory, I might never have gotten breast cancer in 2013, and my menopause journey may have been different.

I remember coming back from Jamaica in 1979 and hating the very idea of fast food. Why, when it took no time to fry two plantains and boil some yam, would I be eating greasy box food? I still think fast food is highly overrated in this time of poverty or cash-rich lifestyles.

The longer you stay away from a place, the more the place seems alien, and the more alien one becomes to it. Frequent visits to Jamaica over the decades were punctuated by the obvious changes in the politics and culture of the 1980s and 1990s, a time of great upheaval in Jamaica, and this impinged on my sense of safety and of belonging to the place. So much so that the idea of settling there again has become a matter for long-term planning and adjustment.

After years of being single and my son now in his late teens, I was looking for a nice bloke, and to celebrate my 40th birthday in April 1998, I hired a small cafe space in Brixton and had a very fancy dinner party, and danced into the wee hours. My cake was a trellis basket design with flowers in beautiful pastel shades, and I was reluctant to cut into it. December that same year I met my second husband at a dinner party. Yes, I like to entertain – a legacy of my Jamaican upbringing.

He wasn't my usual type as he was at least two inches shorter than me, and although he was not an ugly man, he wasn't striking. He was younger than me by about a decade and had a good body – a man who knew hard work, he was very helpful, assisting me all evening with clearing the table and offering to stay behind and help with the washing up. He already had two children back in Jamaica that he adored, and didn't want any more, and I could not have children, I presumed.

I liked him, because we had good conversations; he was very homely, street smart, with good hygiene and lovely teeth. Was it the late bell hooks who said we could fall in love with kindness? He treated me with kindness, and by January the following year, we were an item. My early onset of the menopause meant that I no longer had to worry about an unwanted pregnancy or periods. No need to worry about taking 'birth control', and I was deeply grateful that these worries no longer existed. We had sex like rabbits. I was always moist and the sex was good. The problem was that I had no awareness of the other symptoms of menopause even though I was very emotional, crying almost daily. I recall becoming very depressed and feeling desolate as he was now living in my home. Most of the time I felt vulnerable, some-times with suicidal thoughts, such was my level of despair at the time. Of course, I didn't link my emotional state to early menopause, even though it was out of character. At the time, I thought menopause was just the wearing of hormone patches to make a woman feel less fatigued and the loss of menstruation.

The start of my menopause had also been preceded by a

period of several gynaecological problems to do with having had a coil fitted. 'Controlling birth', as these devices and medications are set up to do, is really a minefield. I regret having had that contraption fitted inside my body as it caused so much pain, infection and trauma to my body. An examination had also revealed endometriosis and some fibroids.

In my early 30s I had surgery for the removal of an ovarian cyst – 'big as a grapefruit', they said. I did not trust these medical professionals, especially after one young woman in a white coat at the hospital told me during the examination that 'I can whip it all out'. This was my uterus she was talking about. She flicked the blonde strands out of her face as she smiled and confidently remarked to her colleagues about removing my reproductive organs. The hospital is a teaching hospital, so I was not sure if she was a student trying to be jolly, but I eased myself off the examination table quickly, got dressed and rushed out, never to return.

I began doing my own research on removal of an ovarian cyst, because 'whip it out' was etched in my brain. She was talking about my reproductive organs, and I was young and married, with only one child. I thought that I might experience more compassion in a hospital dedicated to serving women, so I asked to be referred to the Elizabeth Garrett Anderson and Obstetric Hospital in Euston. The surgeon, the late Dr Boutwood, assured me that I would not lose my ovary. To say that I was petrified is an understatement as I signed the necessary consent forms and simply fretted the whole time. As I was coming around from the anaesthetic, I recall being tapped on my shoulder and told by the surgeon that my ovaries had been left intact. Well, that is what I always thought she had said, because going into surgery I was anxious about losing an ovary. What is worrying is that, since then, every time I have an X-ray or ultrasound of my pelvic area, I get asked about my missing ovary. I had always responded emphatically that it *was* there, because I had been told after surgery that it had not been removed. This reply from me had always been met with silence from the person doing the scan. It had been three decades since the surgery, when it finally dawned on me that it couldn't be there if radiographers couldn't see it. The mind is an interesting organ, I tell you, and we believe what we want to believe. Back then I was plagued by my own naiveté and have had my heart crushed far too many times in one lifetime.

As I am going along the menopause journey, I have had a number of challenges, and at my most recent ultrasound in 2020 to check for tumours in my groin, the nurse said it again – there is only one ovary. So, rather than arguing that it *was* there, and to mask my own feelings of shame at possibly having been lied to, I had a frank discussion with her as she confirmed to me that I was definitely missing an ovary. As I recounted my story, she informed me that ovaries can shrink, too, but if that was the case, my ovary had shrunk a long time ago. I am now wondering if parts of it had been cut away with the cyst, or if anything had indeed been left after that surgery. Had my ovary shrunk, or had the surgeon blatantly lied to me? I concluded that this missing or shrunken ovary may also have contributed to the onset of early menopause or loss of my periods, but what do I know?

My gynaecological problems seemed never-ending. I felt like I was always in stirrups having an examination or a scrape. My pregnancy and labour at 25 years old was fairly uneventful – some projectile vomiting and an aversion to certain foods, with an eight-hour long labour and a tear from birthing. The stitch to the tear seemed to take forever to settle and I think it's disturbed nerve endings because certain sexual positions were never comfortable after that.

Ever since my periods started at around age 12, they had been really heavy. I regularly had a sick note for physical education classes and time off school. Periods were painful, physically debilitating and would cause me to vomit and have diarrhoea at the same time. I was sick for at least three of the seven days of my period, and I bled profusely, so I was looking forward to that time in life when I would have periods no more, and I could indulge my love of white panties all year round, a time when I could enjoy sex without the worry or the risks of using birth control or having an unwanted pregnancy.

I knew nothing of the impact of the menopause on a woman's body, nothing at all. I just wanted to be liberated from all this pain and suffering every 28 days. Plus, I was raised in an environment where sex and pregnancy outside marriage was forbidden and would bring family disgrace. That soon became apparent as I progressed through my early teens. The persistent negative messages about the dangers of 'talking to boys' and 'belly not wanted here', even before I had any comprehension of what they were talking about, left a residue of fear and confusion about sex and procreation in my youth, with no one having ever spoken about it in a beautiful, life-affirming way.

I've since learned that my menstruation need not have

been traumatic to the extent that I experienced it, and this suggests that I was dealing with other psychological and emotional issues at the time. I sure was, but I didn't know anything about period trauma as a teen or young woman.

I was taking hot flashes and night sweats in my stride, and if I was having other symptoms, I had no idea what to look out for. I had responded to a menopause notification in my doctor's surgery and attended a clinic where I was given hormone patches that I wore on my bum. I did not want my new partner to see this sticker on my bum, and when I started to feel unwell and nauseous a few months after wearing them, I put it down to the patch and stopped wearing them. After that I sought out natural herbal remedies, such as herbal teas and supplements.

Recently, a colleague introduced me to conversations on menopause and Black women. It was then that I started to learn more about the menopause, its effects, the wide range of symptoms, physiological changes and so on. This was new to me because I remember hearing my aunties talk about 'the change' but I did not interrogate it, as it seemed something that was of no concern or interest to me, and, of course, I was merely just in earshot. No one ever sat down and explained to me what 'the change' was about. I had no education around it, but I really do think that it's all a part of life and living, part of family and love. It should be discussed openly because it's something that's going to come, isn't it?

I remember hearing adults speaking in hushed tones about children coming from a 'surprise pregnancy' and 'late children', or a 'wash belly child', and about the risk of late pregnancy and whether the child would be disabled in some way. Over the years, I mulled these conversations over in my head to find meaning, and came to the realization that it was because babies were being born at a time when the woman they were gossiping about would normally be going through 'the changes'.

So how do I currently cope with my menopause and/or ageing generally? I definitely have brain fog and the occasional night sweat. I find it futile to fight with brain fog, so I just say 'oops, menopause brain' if I can't remember something and I might do a Google search. I do not commit much to memory, even during the daytime, so if it's important to me, I make a physical note. Electronic Post-it note apps are my lifesaver. It's important for me to be relaxed about it all, but I think I'll have a real problem when I can't remember my PIN for the bank, so to prevent that I've got it written down in code. Remembering passwords is the bane of my life.

My best coping strategy is to understand my limitations and practise self-compassion. I sleep with the window cracked open, as I get my best sleep with that fresh, cool air wafting through the room at night. I sometimes have insomnia, so I simply ride with it, drinking chamomile tea at bedtime and avoiding caffeine during the day. I may read a book, play on my phone, watch TV, meditate, listen to the radio, podcasts or an audiobook story, or relaxing, soothing meditative music. I might even do some breath work or draw on a hypnosis technique that I learned around the time that I first started to experience the menopause. Of course, back then I did not attribute my insomnia to menopause. I also like to visit spas to recharge myself, and at a spa in Shropshire, many years ago, I booked an appointment with a hypnotherapist who took me on a journey that included a lovely Caribbean beach with warm sand – my own place of calm in my mind. Now, 20 years later, I still draw on that hypnosis technique as it always works to put me to sleep. Rest is very important to me; everything works better with a good eight hours of undisturbed sleep.

I remember my late Aunty Myrtle, a passive, gentle soul, submissive to her husband and rarely speaking up at family gatherings. She was a great cook, and her cakes and puddings were so legendary that she never fell short of orders for Cornmeal Pudding, Toto, Rum Cake and Bread Pudding. Aunty Myrtle wore a warm smile and was everyone's favourite family member and neighbour, and even her tenants and boarders all spoke highly of her. But my maternal mother would say that her sister was weak and a pushover who allowed herself to be used by people. I noticed that as Aunty Myrtle aged, she became quite outspoken and vociferous, and even let out the odd swear word. I used to laugh a lot when I visited Jamaica and noticed this difference in her, because the new Myrtle seemed so out of character. She became my ally and advocated for me. When she got upset, she would now refuse to ignore her feelings, and I loved how she was managing her life as a widow after her husband had passed, as he had been much older than her. He had not been a very nice person; even though he had been a good provider financially, he was a real tyrant. I really did like Aunty Myrtle's fresh and outspoken persona, which was brought on by her menopausal symptoms, I suspect.

I have always been fairly opinionated and outspoken, and can have a shrill voice and temper alongside it. Conversely,

I am also inclined to be quiet, too, because I am claiming superiority of intellect or intelligence, or I am just too damn tired. Most importantly, wisdom has taught me that some conversations are not going to end well, and it seems to me that I have been impacted emotionally and physiologically.

What I have learned and continue to experience is that there is so much that I do not know about the menopause. I wonder sometimes if, when my periods had stopped early, the menopausal symptoms had kicked in over a long, extended period, or was I getting the signs of ageing and those of menopause conflated? But I did not age visually because of the early onset of menopause. On reflection, menopause is a period of transition, and I do love the wisdom that comes with ageing; it is priceless – that ability to simply sit back and observe with an inner knowing.

7 Black, Trans and Menopausal

Austen Smith (they/them)

In 2021, I attended the multipart conversation 'Bloody Transitions: Queers Decolonizing Menopause' with moderators M'Kali Hashiki and Syd Yang.[1] In this conversational series, we explored the nuances of sex, gender, race and menopause. In that space, I felt brave enough to experience and reflect on my body *as it is*, and not how it should be.

Menopause stories are often white-washed, drained of colour and texture. The social narrative of menopause is homogenized and misses the opportunity to acknowledge menopause as a human experience. These narratives fail to provide accurate reflections of the experiences of trans and gender non-conforming bodies with uteruses. Gender-expansive Black, Brown and Indigenous people's lives and needs are erased from the linear future by way of exclusion. When we think of menopause, the profile is that of a cis-gender woman above 50. It is implied that 'she' is white,

---

1   www.fiercepassions.com/bloodytransitions

cisgender and heterosexual. But I am a 30-year-old Black, queer, trans-masculine and non-binary person, and I am in menopause. The only narrative I've ever read that reflects Black, queer and trans menopause is the one I am writing.

I began my medical transition in 2016 and had my first surgery in 2018, a total hysterectomy. My body entered surgically induced early menopause. I don't fit the profile of someone who *should* be preparing for menopause, so I wasn't adequately informed or supported. My medical team's performance of progressiveness was spot on. They did everything an ally is 'supposed' to do, but it wasn't authentic, and it didn't meet my standards of care. I needed a warm and inviting environment, trauma-informed and culturally sensitive rapport-building ethics. I needed my physician to trust me the first time that I stated I was confident that I would not regret the procedure and want to be pregnant in the future. I needed the sonographer to not rant and rave about my 'beautiful and textbook uterus and ovaries' during an ultrasound to have those organs removed. I needed educational resources and a co-developed holistic aftercare plan. The aftercare plan would have included trans-inclusive healthcare resources with traditional and non-traditional healing practitioners such as acupuncturists, masseuses and herbalists. My aftercare plan would have included follow-up appointments to track hormone levels and emotional shifts. Quality of care would have looked like compassionate and swift action on behalf of my needs, rather than the minimization of my pain and discomfort. Although my experience did not meet my care standards, it gave me space and time to imagine what a culturally integrated, trans-inclusive, body-positive reproductive healthcare system might look like. For many of my healthcare providers, I was their first trans-masculine patient, which required a lot of free labour on my end to educate the medical professionals in charge of prescribing my meds, putting me under and cutting me open.

One of the main treatments for menopausal management is oestrogen therapy. While I'm happy this option is available for those it serves, it's not viable for trans-masculine and gender non-conforming folks on testosterone replacement therapy. In addition to the lack of medical support and resources, there are very few menopausal support groups that are trans-inclusive. I had never participated in one until I attended 'Bloody Transitions'.

I learned that perimenopause is the transition period a body goes through to prepare for menopause. I also learned that perimenopause is estimated to begin a decade before menopause – although significant racial and ethnic disparities can impact transition start and duration. A multiethnic study specific to cisgender women discovered that Black women enter perimenopause and menopause earlier, have longer transitions and endure worse symptoms.[2] Black women and gender-expansive menopausal experiences are still significantly under-researched, so the general information made available doesn't take historical racialized and gendered medical and systemic violence into account. The menopausal transition is marked by several symptoms, including, but not

---

2   Levine, B. (2022) 'What experts want women of color to know about menopause.' *Everyday Health*, 13 January. Available at: www.everydayhealth.com/menopause/what-experts-want-bipoc-women-to-know-about-menopause, accessed 30 August 2022.

limited to, a decrease in oestrogen, which can cause irregular periods, urinary tract infections (UTIs), hot flashes, heart palpitations, intense premenstrual syndrome (PMS) symptoms, muscle aches, loss of sex drive and difficulty concentrating. While the journey from perimenopause to menopause takes about a decade for age-related transitions, my journey took a little under two hours, which was the time it took the Da Vinci robotic system to remove my uterus and ovaries. The menopause journey is different for *everybody*.

Imagine that for the past 25 years you've taken the same route home every day. This route is optimal and safe. It's so familiar that landmarks along the route have become placement indicators, ways of locating oneself. You don't need a GPS. You've seen the same trees grow and bud and shed every year. One day, there are unexpected blockades on a significant portion of your route, causing you to reroute your process. Now, you must go out of your way to find a new route home. There is no GPS. This scaffolded new route takes significantly longer, with utterly different scenery and unfamiliar landmarks. This route also has wonky traffic patterns with potholes you didn't know to avoid. The are many dead ends. You try to be present with the change, but your patience is wearing thin. You arrive at what should be home, but your house is not there. You are sure you are just lost and need to find the right road. You never find that road, or that home, again. This simplified visual demonstrates when a relatively sudden obstruction along a well-worn path creates infinite possibilities, but going back to the way things were isn't one of those possibilities. I immediately knew that my body, as I formerly knew it, had died. Physiologically, cognitively and emotionally, menopause had remade me. My skin, hair and tastes for certain foods began to change. I was struggling to synthesize information, and my thoughts seemed permanently scrambled. I was being rearranged from the inside out. Words felt hard, and still do. My spirit was somehow more accessible, but the path home, and even the foundation I had come to know as my home, had vanished.

In the beginning, it all felt so overwhelming. I am grateful for my therapist, who was the first to give it a name. In one of our sessions, they reflected on much of what I shared and described the experience as menopause. They invited me to be curious about it, but warned me that much of the content online was anti-Black and gender-restrictive. My therapist then generously offered to do research for me as an act of solidarity, and altered the gender-based language to be gender-neutral during our sessions. Much of the material, resources and communities that focus on menopause erase the narratives of menopausal Black, Brown, Indigenous people of colour, gender-expansive individuals and people who live at the intersection of both. We're here; our stories just don't get amplified. After discovering menopause through my therapist, it was clear to me that quality of care from the medical-industrial complex is not only a want, but also a need. I needed a healthcare team made up of professionals who were sensitive, compassionate and culturally aware enough to prepare me for life beyond the procedure.

Recovery was a slow descent into the pits of menopausal hell, evidenced by the oceanic heatwaves that washed over me day and night. Night-time was awful. I began to dread those beautiful Kentucky sunsets because that was the signal of a sun that would rise inside me. I also experienced severe postoperative complications. I lost significant amounts of blood every day for several months following. The internal wounds had to be cauterized weekly, and the excessive bleeding led to two emergency room visits within the first month. During this time, I wanted my medical team to care more than they were trained to care about bodies, about Black-skinned, trans and gender non-conforming bodies. But the world spun on profusely. Between my body's complications, mundane systemic violence, mediocre healthcare options and the immediate onset of menopause, I became a shell of myself. The modification of my life was business as usual. People were too busy being happy about my transition to notice that I wasn't okay. For a while, I was caught up in their hype. But somewhere in the corner of my heart, grief ached tremendous and silent. Menopause was a renderer, reckoning and mirror, asking: *Are you ready to become?* It was the first of many invitations into a portal of sensuous demise.

According to the organization Being Here, Human, *disenfranchised grief* is 'when the bereaved person's grief does not meet the previously established norms within their culture. This means the person won't receive the support, empathy, and understanding from others they need or desire to metabolize their grief well.'[3]

Black expressions of grief are often restricted and reduced by the limited imagination of white linearity. When we grieve, we're conditioned to do so in socially digestible, respectable ways aligned with the values of whiteness. The mourner's

---

3   www.beingherehuman.com/online-grief-literacy-training

decorum for Black people is to *suck it up*. Make sure no one knows your body produces salt. Whether it be sweat or tears, make it look effortless. So, when I found myself dealing with grief and loss after my first gender-affirming surgery, it felt incredibly isolating. The words needed to describe my experience have yet to be invented. This piece is a thought experiment, exploring with almost-but-not-quite language. I felt that if I went public with the grief of losing something I didn't want to begin with, my grief would be invalidated. It felt as if grieving the loss of a certain relationship with my body brought my transness into question. Mostly because white-dominant trans narratives portrayed in the media necessitate a former self and encourage the complete dis-owning of any part of that former self. These narratives focus solely on sex organs and do not integrate the spiritual or the ancestral, which are core components of Black gender ex-pressions. Still, the conditioning of those narratives resulted in my questioning my own experience and almost made me forget that I am a multitudinous being, capable of missing my uterus from a place of no regrets. Based on how reckless the world is with Black hearts, I couldn't risk it. I stayed inside my shell. Researching about menopause only perpetuated the grief, so I stopped exploring. Asking for the medical attention I needed required me to temporarily suspend my gender expansiveness to pretend to be a woman or trans man in exchange for help. I am neither, so I stopped attending appointments. My world got smaller and smaller. I resorted to hiding from menopause.

Black, gender-expansive beings deserve adequate health-care. We also deserve the time, space and resources to grieve.

We deserve effort from our cisgender and binary-transgender comrades to self-educate, ask questions and learn how to hold space for the reality of complex loss that can come with liberation. Transitioning isn't linear. Transitioning isn't the promise of a blank slate. We need spaces to grieve what was without being gaslit into believing that our grief is regret. My gender-affirming surgeries were some of the kindest and sweetest offerings I ever made at my altar. I'm honoured to be trusted by my benevolent ancestors to transcend systemic binaries of life while I'm still here. There is significant joy in knowing I am doing what I came here to do. In many ways, I am my ancestor.

I bear witness to the deaths I died to live. I grieve that the neurological routes I used to take to some of my most intelligent, brightest contributions are permanently closed. I grieve the electricity surging, hugging the curves of a well-worn road. I grieve the familiarity of my body all while relishing in this sense of freedom that menopause has given me. I celebrate that menopause is a rite of passage that comes with age, and for some, it is a rite of passage that exceeds linear notions of time. I want to see narratives of menopause that honour the biodiversity of human bodies. I want to see a healthcare system evolved by the progress of reproductive rights for all bodies. I invite possibilities from a place of acknowledging that hormones are not gendered until we gender them, that bodies are not gendered until we gender them. Not every woman experiences menopause. Not every woman who experiences menopause is cisgender. Not everyone who experiences menopause is a woman. There is abundant space for Black, queer, trans and gender non-conforming menopausal narratives. I, for one, am counting on the evolution of this topic.

Going through menopause and puberty simultaneously is chaotic and tranquil, sacred and profane. It is linear time collapsing in on itself, folding into a nuance, a crease, a crack that feels novel and unprecedented. I am bending time, merging eldership with the vitality of my youth. My body is a dynamic portal to what is possible, a relic of worlds to come.

8 Manifesting Wellness

Jacqueline Hinds

The menopausal journey is a rite of passage that we face at a significant point in our lives, and for Black women that journey is fraught with many more challenges than the expected symptoms of the change.

As an Emotional Intelligence (EI) coach, I've always immersed myself in its practices and principles and, because of the nature of my work, it was imperative that I kept my finger on the pulse of EI, especially in the working environment. To me, my emotional wellbeing is as essential as the air I breathe. I say this because having spent so much time in a variety of working environments and industry arenas, I've seen discrimination play out in many ways, impacting many people, including myself. I realized early on that I needed to 'step off the planet' and find a space where I could offload the trials and tribulations of my role and the working environment, which, I must admit, had varied gradients of toxicity, depending on where I worked.

More recently, I've been working on a multilateral approach to EI because, to be honest, as a Black person I need insight into how to tap into and top up my knowledge skills and expertise in managing my emotions and understanding others. But I never really gave the menopause or all the symptoms that come with it a second thought. I had always assumed that since I had given birth to my son in my late 40s, 'Madame Menopause' would not be residing with me until I was in my late 60s! How wrong was I on that one!

I had to understand and navigate the landscape of inequalities that Black people must often traverse for career progression and other ventures, goals and aspirations, and the COVID-19 pandemic has amplified the discrimination we face in the workplace. When menopause is added into the equation, and I was going through symptoms of the 'change', I was even more marginalized and not given equitable treatment. Too often, I inadvertently fed into that skewed trope of being a strong Black woman feeling little or no pain, continuing through the battles of life, on little or no sustenance or respite whatsoever. But there came a point where I reclaimed my authority and took ownership of not only my emotions but also how, when and why I responded to indifference, suppression and discrimination within workplaces as I battled and navigated the menopausal journey and landscape.

Reality of the situation

My story centres around my experience of being severely bullied at a senior level in the workplace, and how I used EI to navigate through the highly toxic environment, where I eventually submitted a grievance, which was upheld 100 per cent. All of this was experienced while supporting others, mostly Black women, who were undergoing bullying and harassment while I myself was.

Looking back, I realize that at that juncture in my life, I was going through the perimenopausal journey, as were many of the Black women I was supporting, and my saving grace along that journey was the fact that I was able to put aside my feelings and symptoms to a certain degree, in order for me to fully support and concentrate on others. This was quite cathartic for me as it allowed me to step off the platform and breathe and not think about my situation. It also gave me time to take stock of the game play that I was being drawn into by senior management, and I was able to tap into my EI and effectively assess the situation and not give them what they were trying to provoke – the angry Black woman.

The angry Black woman doesn't exist, but what we do have, like everyone else on this planet, are emotions. Too often as a Black woman I was not afforded the luxury of showing those emotions. Instead, I was ignored, undermined and sidelined and, woe betide if I dare raise any legitimate concerns pertaining to my symptoms or point out differential treatment received against white counterparts. So I felt it would be a good idea to garner some information from other Black women on their own respective menopausal journeys, and gain insight into how they maintained their emotional wellbeing within the workplace or in general. I then had individual conversations with some lovely ladies called Maria, Judith, Susan and Dianne,[1] all of whom are from different

---

1   All names in this chapter have been anonymized.

working backgrounds and ages, all with their own stories to tell of their experiences going through the menopause and the steps they took to safeguard their emotional health and wellbeing.

Overcoming the stigma

Maria never thought about the menopause until she had a conversation with her mother, and this was only after going on a fantastic family holiday in Barbados and not enjoying one bit of it! She had low energy and was anxious, with chronic fatigue, wanting to stay in bed throughout the holiday. At one point her partner thought that she might be pregnant simply because of her symptoms and the way she was behaving. When she got back from holiday, she confided in her mother who was a nurse.

She was surprised when her mother suggested that she was most likely going through the menopause, and that she herself had gone through it at Maria's age, which at the time was 46. Marie admitted that when her mother first suggested that it was the menopause, she laughed and said isn't it what women in their 50s and 60s go through? Her mother went on to say that her menopause symptoms were severe and that she had been on HRT for 10 years! At hearing this, Maria was mortified and said, 'Never in a million years would I have thought that it was the menopause that I was going through.' Maria was a bit like me in thinking that 'Madame Menopause' wouldn't be hitting her any time soon, because she was far too young. There has been a lot of stigma around the menopause, and I suppose in our conversation we were synergized in our thinking of the symptoms, but not only that, we'd both been severely bullied at work while going through our symptoms. For Maria, her fight for justice continues.

Varied impacting symptoms

With the variety of symptoms that occur, not every woman will experience all of them. Some may experience a few, and some none whatsoever – it really is the luck of the draw, or if you are able to glean essential information from your mother. It's funny, though – not all mothers talk to their daughters about their own experiences of going through the menopause. I can't recall my mother mentioning it at all. I can only remember there were times she was so angry, and it seemed about simple things, or it was for nothing at all and just came out of the blue. I didn't know anything about the menopause back then, so it was not something I would follow up on at that juncture.

Now I can only talk about how I'm experiencing my own symptoms, which started to manifest about eight years ago. At first, I paid no attention to what I was experiencing and put it down to me keeping on top of my role at work and supporting others, all while I was being bullied. Oh yes, not to forget I had a family and they needed my time and duty of care too, so self-care was not in the picture then!

I asked all the ladies about their experiences with the symptoms and how they coped and what supplements they took to alleviate the symptoms.

Judith suffered with fibroids, so her periods were quite heavy, but, after an operation and a course of medication to shrink the fibroids, she noticed that her periods, although much lighter, were less regular and that she started to feel warm and agitated quite frequently. She did some research and found out that they were the signs of being perimeno-pausal; she then went full steam into the menopause at the age of 48. She was very sensitive and would get upset very easily, but instead of letting it out, she internalized it, getting offended by the slightest things. Despite that, she was not interested in taking HRT and sought out natural products to help alleviate her symptoms and emotions.

Susan and Dianne were very much on the ball and took affirmative action with their symptoms. Susan had hot flashes and mood variations, so her doctor suggested HRT. But she chose to look at natural remedies instead, which worked wonders for her, alleviating the symptoms completely over a period of time. She now only takes them a couple of times a week as opposed to daily. She also took some time away from work to get herself together and to tackle the overwhelming feelings and symptoms she was experiencing.

Dianne had started experiencing the symptoms of the menopause about three years ago, and noticed that she was reacting to certain situations in a way that was unlike her true self. She would often self-reflect and wonder why she had reacted the way she did, and that led her to research on her symptoms and behaviour and to conclude that she was going through the menopause. Dianne is very much into natural herbal products and would venture to see the 'Herbsman' who had a shop in South London, where she would purchase all the 'back home' herbs and remedies that were not available in our high street shops.

Feelings of oppression

It was not easy keeping my emotions in check when I was miserable. Trust me, there were days I felt I just wanted to pull the duvet over my head and wait for the day to end. The symptoms had me under siege and hijacked all my sense and reasoning, replacing it with low mood, lack of confidence and general apathy. To make things worse, it was somewhat amplified by being discriminated against in the workplace.

I was curious to find out whether any of the women I spoke to were given any kind of support or signposting to networks or services they could access to support them with queries or questions they may have regarding their symptoms and general feelings during the menopause.

Judith said that her symptoms were exacerbated, and as a Black manager she felt quite sensitive and slightly paranoid while being constantly terrorized by staff, because, as their manager, she would request that things be done in a certain way. This experience made her question and overthink everything she did in her role, making her feel that she wasn't allowed to have or show her emotions. No form of support was given to her, but her white counterparts were given support and time off.

Maria wasn't given any form of support; instead, she was bullied and victimized to the point that she had to be signed off by her doctor on long-term sick leave, and, after being back for a couple of weeks, was signed off sick again. The onslaught was horrendous, and the ill treatment took its toll time and time again. She has since left the organization and has taken them to tribunal for sex and disability discrimination, victimization, management bullying and harassment and stress at work. Her case has drawn a lot of attention and she is looking forward to it concluding so that she can get her life back after being subjected to a perpetual cycle of oppression.

How does culture fit in?

When it comes to being treated equitably and with compassion, Black women are the most disrespected out of all the female humans on this planet. Sounds harsh, doesn't it? Well, I'm not wrong there. Our culture and race as Black women inadvertently places a bullseye on our backs, which is unjustified and unwarranted.

Having to wear an emotional mask is tiring, and in speaking to the women, I get the sense that in the workplace, to safeguard their emotional health and wellbeing, they have worn that mask of pretence that everything is fine and nothing untoward is brewing. The thing is, as a Black woman, I was not even allowed to be my authentic self in the workplace. I have had to justify my very presence on this planet, not forgetting the comments that come around how we dress, the food we eat and our myriad of fantastic and versatile hairstyles. Culture certainly plays a big part in the discrimination Black women face along their respective menopausal journeys.

When it comes to emotions, many Black women like me do not like to show them. This could be something that has been ingrained within us culturally, but it also feeds into the misrepresented narrative that Black women are strong and can take a lot of pressure, and still manage to under-take our roles with few or no problems. Even when I was trying to be reasonable and calm, trying to ignore the slings and arrows that workplace bullies were firing at me, there was this persistent provocation from oppressors who, again, wanted to provoke the angry Black woman to justify the harsh, unwarranted mistreatment, victimization and bullying that they have been subjecting us Black menopausal women to over prolonged periods of time. This treatment will almost certainly have an adverse effect on anyone's emotional health and wellbeing.

What did I do to safeguard myself?

By understanding and adopting the practices and prin-ciples of EI, you can really gain insight into others' behaviour and mindsets. Emotional resilience (ER) is key to supporting myself as a Black menopausal woman having faced challenges in the workplace, social setting, home or church.

For clarity, I'd like to explain that ER is 'the process of adapting well in the face of adversity, trauma, tragedy, threats or even significant sources of stress – such as family or rela-tionship problems, serious health problems or workplace and financial stressors'[2] – basically, being able to bounce back from difficult situations.

The three key components of ER I adopted along my journey were very much like a formula:

$$SI + EI + EM = ER$$

---

2   APA (American Psychological Association) (2014) *The Road to Resilience.* Washington, DC: APA, para. 4.

Sensory intelligence (SI) is the understanding of how your senses unconsciously respond to the environment to impact how you live, learn and work. Emotional intent (EI) is the ability to care about your dominant emotions enough to let feelings come forth and follow it through, and emotional management (EM) is the ability to be aware of, and constructively handle, both positive and challenging emotions.

My emotional wellbeing is just as valuable to me as it is to anyone else. As a Black woman, it was imperative that I adopted a more emotionally intelligent approach in dealing with my menopausal symptoms, as well as the challenges I faced within the workplace. I had to deal with conflict in an effective and resolution-driven way, and although I couldn't change the way I was treated by others, I certainly felt adequately equipped and empowered to challenge the status quo and command the respect I deserved but had long been denied.

I see my menopausal journey as a rite of passage, and it is down to us to impart the knowledge around the symptoms and effects they have on our emotional health and wellbeing to others, especially Black women and girls, because they are our future Black leaders and professionals of tomorrow. Knowledge is power, so they say, but it is only powerful and potent when it is shared with others who can take this dissemination of information forward, progressing it toward loftier heights and achievements. This is a charge to all women, to encourage them to continue to share their stories and journeys with others. In doing so, this will help them along their own respective journeys.

9 The Mask of Professionalism

Me, Menopause and Work
Sandra Wilson

I want to highlight that this is my story, and it is important for me to mention this because everyone has their own unique path. When I commenced my writing, it was the first time that I was reflecting on my journey of work and why it has been so important to me as a woman and the way that it affected how I experienced the menopause.

Background

For the many generations of women within my family, work, whether it be as an entrepreneur, self-employed or as an employee, has afforded us the means to have our own money and enabled a level of independence, choice and socialization. In my mother's and aunties' case, it provided them with a voice to make decisions both within the home and at work. When I was a child, my mum used to say, 'If you have to ask a man for money to buy your own knickers, you are giving him power. You must have your own money.' She believed work was a means of survival and independence for women like us, and by 'us' she meant Black women.

My mother took great pride in herself; she would visit the hairdresser once every two weeks for the obligatory shampoo-and-set, shopped for clothes from Marks & Spencer, which was a big deal in those days, and during the latter years of her life graduated to shopping at the Harrods and Selfridges sales. She would always make it known that she paid for those treats with her own money, and if there was ever an argument between my mum and dad about her personal spending, I could hear her say, 'It's my money which I have worked for. I have not asked you to pay for it.'

Growing up at home, I either overheard or was included in conversations about the marginalization of African and Caribbean people in the UK, and my mum, who was a nurse, and dad, a motor mechanic, spoke freely about the multiple layers of discrimination that they faced because of their race and class, and, in my mum's case, her gender – this layered discrimination is now commonly known as 'intersectionality'. My parents had a strong work ethic, and earning money gave them a sense of independence while raising a family. I remember being told at a very young age that, as a Black woman, success in the UK would not be easy, and that I needed to work harder and do better to even get a seat at the table. My mum believed it was important for me to know how to put on 'the mask of professionalism', to be the best at what I did, and to never be complacent. In her eyes, there was no room for vulnerability.

I was always mindful of what I shared with people because my parents told me to 'keep your business to inside the home', and especially when it came to women's issues such as menstruation – I was told never to discuss it outside the home, and especially with men. My parents told me stories about the times that they had been let down by people because they had shared family matters with someone outside the home.

The mask of professionalism

I give this backdrop from my past to emphasize that work for the females in my family was considered integral to having a level of independence and freedom, and that as a Black female I was also taught that it was important to be at the top of my game. My dad used to say that 'being white was a qualification in itself', and he would warn me about the inequalities I would face because of my race and gender. Growing up, I subconsciously strived for perfection while at the same time living with the changes in society and hearing the mantra 'women can have it all' and the term 'strong Black woman', which I suspect were the dominant phrases at the time.

Even after the breakdown of my parents' marriage when I was 12, their strong messages stayed with me, and when I got married at 21, much to their delight, I had already started my public sector career. As a trainee committee clerk, I found myself within a system that was, and still is, very much underpinned by patriarchy, and continues to be predominately snow-white at senior level. I thank my parents for explaining to me about the mask of professionalism because it has served me well.

While at work, I met a wonderful new friend, and to protect identities, I will call her Margaret – she was 20 years my senior, very sophisticated, always professional and on point. By 'on point', I mean she was shit hot! She knew her stuff, was highly respected by everyone and had a charismatic presence and an air of authority about her. I remember thinking that if I was lucky enough to get to that age, I wanted to be like her. But then there came a time when Margaret had a long period of sick leave, and when she finally returned to work, I noticed that although she was beautifully dressed, she was clearly not herself – there was something missing: the sparkle in her eyes had disappeared.

Talking to Margaret was my first in-your-face real encounter with menopause. She confided in me that she had been menopausal for over four years, had managed the symptoms using HRT (hormone replacement therapy), but had to come off it for a while because of an operation. She stated that she was feeling 'like shit' and would have to leave work if the symptoms continued. She had told her manager about the operation but chose not to mention the menopause because she did not want to be judged as 'old and past it'. She felt that women's issues should be kept out of the workplace, even though she was finding it a challenge to cope. She also wore 'the mask of professionalism'. She often spoke about not wanting to give up work because of the importance of having her own money, and she was looking forward to the pension that she had worked hard to accumulate. Eventually, she was given a lower dose of HRT, which she said made her feel more like herself. Reflecting on that time, and knowing how much I hate the idea of not being in control, I decided when I eventually went through the menopause, that I would also use HRT.

My chats with Margaret were my first introduction to menopause, and I did not think about it again as I was in a different season of my life, busy being a wife and a mother, and juggling a career. As time passed, I became aware of other women experiencing the menopause, and I certainly wasn't prepared for its arrival.

Being scared

To be honest, I am not sure when the perimenopause started for me, but a particular incident in 2015 highlighted a pivotal moment in my working life. I had always prided myself on having a good memory, but I noticed that I was having trouble remembering stuff, and that I was sometimes confused, depressed and feeling like I was losing my grip on life. At home, Lloyd, my husband, said that I was becoming challenging to live with, snapping at him for nothing and often repeating myself. Both Emma and Laura, my daughters, echoed this. I cried a lot in secret, but one day I cried at work, which caused a bit of a stir with my colleagues – my professional mask was slipping. I was not in a good place, but I did not link it to the menopause because I was not experiencing hot flushes, which I had known to be one of the classic symptoms, so in my mind I was simply losing it. I tried desperately to hold on to who I was, but I was becoming extremely vulnerable – I was scared.

During 2015, after a particularly long day at work and what seemed like a mega commute home – you know those commutes, when you just about get on to the Tube or bus and people are breathing all over you (this was pre-pandemic times). I arrived home and noticed that I was sweating profusely, soaked through to my outer coat and feeling very much under the weather – my body and head were in agony. I took a long shower, thinking that I had clearly overdone it at work, but something was clearly wrong with my body, and maybe I did not realize it, or maybe I did not want to admit it to myself, but I was in a scary place. When Lloyd asked me if I was okay, I did that thing, 'yep, I am fine, just a little tried', but when we retired to bed, I got an overwhelming feeling in the pit of my stomach that all was not well.

During that night, I went to the washroom and returned to bed feeling dizzy, hot, clammy and confused, and I actually thought I was dying. I cannot recollect much from that night, only that I ended up in hospital not able to walk straight, dizzy, confused and being physically sick. After several tests, I was diagnosed with vertigo – an imbalance in the ear – and for the first time in my life I was signed off work for a significant period of time.

The consultation

During one of my regular GP visits, I was referred to an onsite specialist in women's issues and had an unexpected extended consultation of 45 minutes that included an explanation of what the menopause was, advice on diet and the choices available to me. At the end of the consultation I opted for HRT, a referral to a CBT (cognitive behavioural therapy) specialist, and was recommended for a free diet and exercise regime. I thoroughly enjoyed the experience of therapy, and despite breaking the golden rule of not telling my business to a stranger, it was nice to have the weekly calls and to work through my issues in a confidential space. I needed all the help I could get.

I was concerned about whether I would be able to work again, and my independence is very important to me. Thankfully, when I returned to work, I changed to a different role, adjusted my working hours, and the counselling really helped. My memory returned, although not at the same level. I also had more energy and was coping. Unfortunately, I have since developed anxiety, which I had never experienced prior to the menopause, and which is exacerbated when I am stressed, so I have developed a number of coping strategies.

The workplace

When I returned to work, I was amazed to find a menopause support network of women of all backgrounds sharing their stories and challenges. The sharing of stories and advice was uplifting. We had lots of conversations on a range of topics – we spoke about our collective desire to maintain our professionalism, of wearing the corporate mask, about the lack of understanding of what was happening to our bodies, the secrecy and the shame of menopause and the diverse list of symptoms, as well as how we could influence change in the workplace. The Menopause Network provided a safe haven to be able to tell my story without being judged.

One of the great benefits of the network was the guidance it produced for managers, and the information that became accessible for all staff. Thankfully, many more organizations are incorporating policies to support all those impacted by the menopause journey. What I found is that the challenge now is to hear the voices from people who are still underrepresented within this space. This has motivated me to share my story with diverse groups of women, especially those from the African and Caribbean communities. There are times when I share my journey and someone will say that they have similar symptoms but did not even consider that they could be menopausal. I have also supported others who try to keep it together and have not wanted to seek help because of the historical lack of trust that exists within the Black community when it comes to the medical profession.

My new norm

Menopause has helped me to be more myself. I no longer choose to wear the professional mask at all, I wear clothes that are comfortable and reflect my cultural heritage, and I openly talk about menopause in the workplace because I no longer see it as taboo, or exclusively a women's issue – it impacts everyone. I am open about my upbringing as it gives context to why I am the way that I am.

It is fair to say that the time is right for being outspoken. We have all been through a pandemic, and there is more focus today on the injustices and divisions in society, like the Back Lives Matter and the #MeToo movements, which have provided platforms for open discussions. I am now better able to use my voice to discuss the previously whispered conversations, the unmentionables, and if my parents were alive today, I think they would agree that this is the time to talk.

The dates when my peri-, or, indeed, menopause, started are still very unclear in my head because I believe there was a denial that something was wrong, which stemmed from my belief that I would no longer be able to work – I feared dependence on someone else, being ill and vulnerable. For too long, it was easier to wear the crumbling professional mask rather than seek help, but it was the final acknowledgement in hospital that I was too sick to work that led me to make the valuable changes to my life. I returned to work with a renewed focus and more of my authentic self – I started putting me first. I am still on that journey and there are still numerous challenges, but I now have the tools and the community to support me when I need it.

Menopause has impacted every aspect of my life and I have had to systematically make changes to accommodate this new me. I now view myself and my health through a holistic lens, and realize that some of my old belief systems no longer serve me. I live more in the moment and with purpose, and I am thriving. I manage my anxiety, work a shorter week and take regular mini holiday breaks away to reflect. I have invested in a fitness regime and have changed my diet and, most importantly, I bask in the love of my family and close friends and give thanks. To reflect, I would say that menopause is just another season in life, and it has enabled me to drop a lot of the baggage associated with my past and to live a more authentic life where it is okay to be vulnerable at times and to ask for help.

10 Mama K's Ghana Experience

Mbeke Waseme

Ghana in West Africa has a population of 32 million.[1] Approximately 49 per cent of them are female, with an average age of the menopause being 48.5 years. As someone who has lived and worked in Ghana for a while, I wanted to find out more about the experience of menopause in this beautiful country, and compare it with my own personal experience, having spent most of my life in the UK.

This is an important public health topic, but the research in Ghana seems limited and sketchy. Does this speak to the lack of importance that this crucial change in a woman's life is given, or is this another area of Ghanaian society that is known and accepted and 'not made a fuss about'?

I initially set out to do a short questionnaire but had difficulty getting people to respond, which was frustrating. On reflection, I think the reluctance was mainly because menopause is not often spoken about – not because of some

---

1 www.worldometers.info/world-population/ghana-population

social taboo, but because the women just get on with their lives. Girls will grow up hearing about their menstrual cycle and they will be prepared for this, and many will be shown how to manage themselves and their bodies when their menstrual flow begins. In their more mature years, this does not happen and women are not prepared for the menopause, so I spoke with men and women in a local store, asking them what they knew about the menopause. Over 50 per cent knew nothing and the other 50 per cent said that it was a time when women change – they go a little crazy; many lose their memories; some have serious hot sweats; some become witches.

I then had a chat with Mama K about her personal experience, and here is what she told me.

To be very honest, I did not know how or when the 'less-talked-about menopause moment' would catch up with me. In fact, I expected it to finally appear perhaps in my mid-60s, but here I was, somewhere at the brink of my late 50s, experiencing some signs. My first realization of it was in the area of the changes I experienced in my flow cycle. I realized that my monthly flows were not very consistent; the period and the quantity of flow had decreased immensely.

However, I had not had any prior education or advice regarding the way a woman approaching this experience would be and how she was expected to handle menopause. Yes, sometimes I had cramps in my lower abdomen. It felt like something was pulling me from within, but I never really attributed it to menopause alone since I was already dealing with an ulcer. I had heard myths surrounding medications that could help, yet I was not interested to know what they were. In all sincerity, I was never particular about eating any kind of food and neither did I take any special medication. I ate my favourite staple foods and most of them were fufu, rice and yams, just because I enjoyed eating them.

What I can recall vividly was that my sister, who was visiting Ghana from the States, introduced me to 60 plus capsules, a dietary supplement for women aged 60 or above.

I must say that it took the intervention of some of the ladies in the health sector of my local church to hold a discussion around the topic before I started paying close attention to this part of my life. After I had come to terms with the menopause, thanks to our women's group, I bounced back to being less anxious. I guess I had come to embrace the fact that it was a stage in life, and I was happy to have experienced it in my lifetime.

This is the experience that many Ghanaian women have, and with over 70 per cent of the population being Christian, it is understandable that a church group would provide the information and support for women going through the menopause.

At the beginning, I will say that I was oblivious to the changes in my body. I had been working for a greater part of my life, and just like most women in Ghana do, I did not pay close attention to the things that matter.

I started experiencing and noticing the changes when I first observed the irregularities in my monthly flow.

I also noticed that they were either a heavy flow or a low flow; other times the flow came too early or too late, but definitely very different from the normal. I will admit that, regardless of all these changes, I never visited a physician to complain. I just accepted that it was something normal, something that happens to every woman, especially women my age.

Girls' minds are prepared toward menstruation, but no one is prepared towards menopause. There are women who may not want to drive and choose to spend more time alone, and who have been described as 'continually complaining of illness and feeling moody and depressed'; there are others who have thinning hair, swollen ankles, weight gain, bloating, hot flushes and reduced levels of energy. But they do not know how to cope.

Sometimes friends and family get impatient with the women who are experiencing these changes, and in some remote communities, when the changes have been so extreme that it leaves them disorientated and vastly different to their usual selves, they are thought to be witches with supernatural powers.

Mama K and I went on to discuss a lot more about menopause in Ghana, and I was enlightened.

Most women in Ghana grow up in an environment where their lives include regular squatting. Crouching or squatting is a standard position that Ghanaians take when they are performing a wide range of activities that require them to be close to the ground. Sometimes, instead of sitting on a chair, they will squat when having general conversations.

These activities of crouching and squatting help to increase their bone density, improve their mobility and strengthen their core muscles, and they are also known to help alleviate urinary incontinence. So it is very apparent that Ghanaian women are deriving benefits from their cultural lifestyle.

Many Ghanaian women also do a lot of walking, carrying and balancing things on their head, and these activities are known to aid posture as they brace the body as though it were a straight column. Carrying weights when walking means that the women are making their bodies work harder, which helps them to burn extra calories, and the weight that they carry on their heads engages and strengthens the muscles that are deep in their necks. These Ghanaian women, without really speaking about it or maybe even realizing, are strengthening their spine and posture as well as supporting their urinary health.

During the menopause, the production of oestrogen in the body is reduced. Up until this point, oestrogen has made the monthly menstrual cycle possible, and with the body no longer producing this hormone, the body's thermostat slowly stops working. The results are a range of symptoms such as hot flushes, night sweats, anxiety and a low interest in sex. I suspect, however, that there may also be something in the Ghanaian diet that lends itself to a less extreme experience of the menopause.

Are there benefits to be derived from a diet that is rich in yams? Could eating yams on a regular basis affect menopause symptoms? In Ghana, yams are eaten regularly in a variety of ways – for example, fried yam chips, roasted or boiled yam to accompany stews, candied yam, yam porridge and many other dishes. Yams are special to menopause because they contain oestrogen – the same oestrogen that the body produces less and less of during the menopause. In Ghana, a cream made of yam relieves the symptoms of menopause and is offered as an alternative to the allopathic, clinically produced oestrogen cream. While the research is inconclusive on yam cream, there are many who use it because oestrogen does naturally occur in yams.

Another key part of the Ghanaian diet is local fermented foods such as banku (a dish made of fermented corn and cassava dough) and kenkay (a sourdough dumpling made from fermented corn), which is very popular and widely eaten. You can buy it on the street, at the market and in restaurants, and it is also made at home. These foods are made of complex carbohydrates that are rich in vitamins A, C, E, K and B; they help to regulate blood sugar, lower blood pressure and contain high levels of fibre. These foods do not have a strong taste on their own, so they are usually eaten with beans, fish, meat, avocado and pepper sauce – they are generally part of a 'healthy' diet.

Some women use prekese fruit as a supplement, which is known for its healing benefits. It is used in the bath, boiled or added to food. Apparently, it is used for managing diabetes, blood pressure and glucose levels, and it also provides nutrients that the body needs after childbirth to restore blood loss and to help in lactation.

Women's bodies incorporate the benefits of these experiences that begin from when they are small children, and even those women who are in the low socioeconomic sectors have these cultural elements as part of their regular lives. But speaking with Mama K, it was evident that the lifestyles and dietary paths of socioeconomic groups in Ghana may impact how they experience the menopause later in their life.

Unfortunately, some of the women, especially those who are climbing the social ladder and suddenly arrive in the middle, are keen to adopt a Western way of life, so they shun and change some or all of their traditional practices that have been incorrectly associated with 'poverty', 'a backward lifestyle' and being 'bush'. Local foods are exchanged for foreign foods such as pizza, takeaway fried chicken and noodles, walking and crouching are exchanged for sitting in chairs and cars, for bending down from the waist with their legs straight, and valuable time spent outdoors increasing vitamin D uptake is exchanged for time under the fan or with the air conditioning.

I am grateful to Mama K for her time in sharing her experience of this important subject. I conclude that it is important for this subject to be discussed so that women can be prepared through public health promotions. If the opportunity presents itself, I would like to go into villages across Ghana to get more information about how the menopause is perceived and supported.

11 Is HRT Really Necessary?

Asma-Esmeralda Abdallah-Portales

Generally, menopause is when you haven't had a period for 12 consecutive months, and postmenopause is the time after that, but the majority of people refer to postmenopause as menopause. Perimenopause is when the body is transitioning to menopause, and some people can have symptoms as early as in their 30s, but do now know what is happening to their bodies and look for answers of their ill feelings elsewhere.

Taboos around the menopause keep it from being discussed, but slowly knowledge is being passed on to younger generations. Right now, the topic is quite trendy, and the narrative is that we are meant to be strong, not vulnerable. I think that is one of the reasons why menopause is not talked about more, and the stigma of becoming an 'old lady' could make it difficult to face.

Often, we are seen (and see ourselves) as less attractive when starting on this phase of our lives. Also, not being able to reproduce has a connotation of lesser value and worth in a society dominated by patriarchal views of exploitative and extractive systems of capitalism. For some, we are merely seen as birthing machines. I would rather see menopause taught appropriately in schools in biology or sex education, with information provided in a more respectful way and with more quality data. I would also advocate normalizing contact with gynaecologists from an early age to help with the fear associated with menopause at a later stage in life.

Not all women give birth, and a few may sail right through the years from their first menstruation, without many obstacles, to an uncomplicated menopause. No cramps and no hot flashes – the best-known symptoms. But everyone has a different experience because the changes don't just occur through hormones – body weight can fluctuate, skin tissues will age and wrinkles will appear – but these don't all happen at the same time and speed for everyone. This is why I decided to let it go on naturally, and that I would be better without Botox.

I think my menopause started when I turned 50 and went on until I was 65, and every now and then I continue to get sudden hot flashes. I remember how unexpected they were at first, and how embarrassing it was when I started the menopause. Notably, I started having migraines when I was 15 and knew that they had something to do with my menstrual cycle and my metabolism, and I always thought that these migraines would subside during menopause. But no, unfortunately, the migraines still come up periodically. Thankfully, I can say they are not as frequent any more. High blood pressure and migraines are my worst menopause symptoms, and the migraines I suffered that have accompanied me since my teenage years mean that I have had to manage and cope with pain all my working life. I would turn up for work despite being ill for fear of taking too many days off due to stringent sick leave regulations and having to earn a living to bring up my six children.

I went through all possible and known tests, but the real cause of these migraines has never been diagnosed. I have spent many years taking very strong tablets, sumatriptan being the only one that kept me going when the pain was unbearable. I knew that these strong drugs were addictive and could cause people to function in a daze, in a drugged state, so I eventually stopped taking them for fear of the side effects. I am so glad that I did, because as I am getting older, the strong migraine headaches are slowly subsiding, even though I cannot clearly say what the reason for this relief is.

Is taking HRT really necessary?

I was offered oestrogen tablets when I went to my gynaecologist, but I had made up my mind that I would not take them. When I read the prescription leaflet of the pills that I was practically forced to buy, I was shocked that it said that it could increase my risk of having breast cancer. That then confirmed some suspicions I have about certain pharmaceutical products. So instead, I decided to use alternatives. My research, 20 years ago, brought me to the herbal medicine of red clover, and I was so happy because I had sucked the sweetness out of the red clover plant as a child in the German countryside, and remembered my connection to this herb. So, for many years, I bought pills of red clover online and I believe they helped to alleviate the negative symptoms of my menopause to a great extent. I did not really 'suffer' the effects from hot flashes, but I do remember the mood swings that I treated solely with the help of herbal teas. I have always consumed lots of teas, but at that time I drank a lot of milk thistle tea, alchemilla tea, spearmint and peppermint tea as well as gingko and red clover teas.

I had also read some literature that spoke about the Japanese experience of adding soy proteins and soybean to foods to lessen the symptoms and maybe even eliminate many effects that are attributed to the menopause. My understanding is that this is because soy isoflavones have an effect on the thyroid function and that soy is an oestrogen mimicker. Even though I know that there are Asian cultures that do not even have a word for menopause because it doesn't exist in their language, I started cooking with soy sauce, especially vegetables, and used it more and more in my meals.

I also found other natural remedies to alleviate the accompanying symptoms of the menopause, such as diosgenin, extracted from wild yams, which is now available in tablet form as a menopause supplement. Thyroid-related diseases such as Graves' disease are twice as likely to affect Black women than white women, and ginger, turmeric and seaweed such as kelp are also considered to be natural remedies to help with problems of an underactive thyroid, one of the glands that produces hormones and therefore helps to keep them balanced. Nutritionists have recommended increasing selenium, which is a trace element that plays a part in thyroid hormone metabolism, and there are many foods that contain selenium such as tuna, turkey, Brazil nuts and grass-fed beef.

I also read that Black woman can experience hormone

imbalances due to excessive use of hair relaxers, root stimulators and anti-frizz products that contain almost 70 chemicals identified so far, which are known toxins to the human body and affect their endocrine system.[1] Is it any wonder that Black women are more likely than white or Hispanic women to suffer from disorders related to the endocrine system or their hormonal system?

The onset of my menopause came with high blood pressure (hypertension),[2] and before that I mainly had low blood pressure. In the years preceding menopause, the body's oestrogen and progesterone production decreases and testosterone production increases, which has numerous effects on the bloodstream as oestrogen and progesterone imbalances can cause blood vessels to expand and constrict sporadically. Well, this changed my life drastically as I have been taking beta-blockers ever since. I wish I had known about the symptoms of perimenopause and the menopause and the way in which the entire body responds and reacts to it – for example, I strongly believe that one of the best ways for me to deal with hypertension would have been to get the hypothalamus in balance as it helps control blood pressure by producing vasopressin, an antidiuretic hormone, which affects the kidneys' production of urine. More vasopressin means less urine output, which results in higher blood volume and increases blood pressure. Had I known that before, I would have taken greater precautions. I really wish I could

---

1   https://thyroidproblemsdoctor.com/black-women-harmed-by-toxins-in-hair-relaxants; https://thyroidproblemsdoctor.com/thyroid-hormones-cycle
2   Sandra Y (2021) 'Does menopause cause high blood pressure.' Menopause Talk, 17 September. Available at: www.menopausetalk.net/does-menopause-cause-high-blood-pressure, accessed 31 August 2022.

have had someone to speak to about this issue at the time, as I certainly would have had a much healthier and easier life.

I have been taking medication to stabilize my blood pressure and even had to undergo a test at a dialysis centre. The doctor told me that I would probably have to increase the doses of my medication and would most likely end up receiving haemodialysis three times a week. I was devastated! I certainly did not want to have this experience at all! So I have been trying to find natural remedies to reduce my blood pressure ever since, including reducing my salt consumption and using grapefruit, honeydew melons and mistletoe (tea and drops), garlic and hawthorn – anything to keep myself away from more medication and potentially sinister interventions.

Sexuality

I have heard that sexual desire might wane or go away completely during or after the menopause, and that most times it returns. But maybe when it returns, it does so in a different way, because for me, meeting the right person to arouse my desire was vital, and to experience intimacy was important. Sexuality for me is a form of communication and communion and the sharing of nature in gratitude. By listening to my body, nature showed me many times what it needed to be sensually satisfied. Masturbation is still a subject that is generally avoided and stigmatized, and there are so many who do not know what their own vagina looks like, let alone know and talk about the feelings and sensations connected with their own needs. My sexuality was affected by vaginal dryness, and I remember having days when a strong itching sensation would drive me crazy. Had I known that it had to do with vaginal dryness, I would not have been so embarrassed in many instances. Really, it is so easy to keep your vagina moisturized, which helps to prevent some of the severe pain during sexual intercourse that is caused by the dryness and soreness.

Testosterone and fluidity in sexual preferences with the onset of the menopause

I haven't started to grow a beard. In some cultures, it is seen as sexy for women to have a moustache, on others any hair growth is seen as an unwanted nuisance, but some happily embrace their facial hair, even without gender transitioning. As for me, I am certain that my menopause triggered my need to come out as a bisexual and/or lesbian woman. From discussions I have had, it seems that there are a lot of women who experience a greater attraction to their own sex during the menopause, but who are afraid to address the issue publicly. It became a personal necessity for me to come out, and I am glad most of my family accepted me as I am. I have been bisexual since my teenage days, but my mother has never really accepted me – but that's a different story. I wish bisexuality was not as stigmatized as it is.

The Cuban experience

Although Cuba is a relatively poor country, it has a very efficient and free healthcare system for its citizens. The state manages to provide access to medical doctors and surgeries on a local level in all communities for the entire population. When it comes to menopause, the health authorities have made changes, and there have been significant changes in conditions such as osteoporosis, weight management, arterial hypertension and breast cancer. But social and socioeconomic challenges mean having to develop different coping strategies during these times of bodily change. This is not just a Cuban issue; it is a global problem. But in Cuba, where there is an ongoing situation of food shortages and scarcity of certain medicines, many women resort to taking alternative or herbal medicines.

In Cuba, climacterium (the mental and physical reproductive changes that happen during all stages of the menopause) and the symptoms of insomnia and hot flashes, changes in body shape, which can increase the risk of diabetes and cardiovascular problems, irregular menstrual cycles, osteoporosis and vaginal dryness are seen as a naturally occurring event that begins with the menopause, typically around the age of 45–50, although it is different for every woman. Since life expectancy for women in Cuba is now approximately 80, it is estimated that generally women can live about 30 years in a postmenopausal period. Cuban women are generally told to exercise, refrain from taking toxic substances, develop healthy eating habits to avoid obesity and high blood pressure, control cholesterol and risk factors for osteoporosis and, if required, to consider HRT (hormone replacement therapy).[3]

---

3 Ministry of Public Health (Cuba) (2019) 'Menopause, illness or natural?' 18 October [in Spanish]. Available at: https://salud.msp.gob.cu/menopausia-enfermedad-o-naturalidad, accessed 31 August 2022.

Mental health

Emotional wellness during the menopause is a huge subject, and apart from the symptoms mentioned above, sadness and crying a lot are commonly reported. We are often told in Cuba to use natural remedies to help with menopause mental health, such as St John's wort and Bach flower essence, as they can lessen, help to overcome or prevent swinging moods or depression. I personally recommend the nurturing of our women's circles so that we are empowered to speak up and talk about the dark moments we may encounter during our menopause.[4]

> Caring for myself is not self-indulgence, it is self-pres-ervation, and that is an act of political warfare. (Audre Lorde[5])

I personally believe that this quote from Audre Lorde has been appropriated by many people and misused for their own purposes – from promoting interior decorations to golf leisure as radical self-care. But the fact that we are able to discuss mental health more openly is largely due to the courageous activism and struggle of Black women drawing our attention to anger, strength and racism as aspects of pressure that can trigger mental health issues, and not only during menopause.

---

4   Spicer, A. (2021) '"Self-care": how a radical feminist idea was stripped of politics for the mass market.' *The Guardian*, 21 August. Available at: www.theguardian.com/commentisfree/2019/aug/21/self-care-radical-feminist-idea-mass-market, accessed 31 August 2022.

5   Lorde, A. (2017) *A Burst of Light and Other Essays*. Long Island, NY: Ixia Press.

Spiritual growth and the wisdom of the older woman

The real mystery of the menopause for me has always been the beauty of the maturity of the older woman. Instead of fearing the wrinkles of age and marks of experience on my skin, I have always been looking forward to becoming and being an older woman. I admired the elegance and poise of older women from a young age. The power, experience and wisdom we hold is what has actually shielded us from the evils of patriarchy and its unjust and unequal treatment since ancient past history through to contemporary times. Even the burning of supposed witches has not been able to lessen our resilience and strength as we occupy slightly more than half of the world's population. I remember that every time a new woman is born.

Becoming my true self and being free to be me started with the menopause, and even though finding out how I want to be as this new woman can be a challenge, I embraced my age, experience and wisdom that I acquired leading up to and during the menopause as an asset. Having children or preferring to remain childless should not take away from how you want to protect yourself in the world, and living in authenticity becomes so much easier after the menopause. I have chosen to live my life in the way that I identify as having centred myself despite what my surrounding environments might want to tell me, and I try to enjoy the sensations. I let the hot flashes burn away the old beliefs about women; while they may last only a few seconds, I let the waves come and go to strengthen my self-worth. I let the menopausal transformation take place and let the fire die out in the end.

The menopause is meeting our demons and hidden aspects every day as mortality becomes a feasible thing on the horizon, and as the body is withering down, death becomes a reality, so facing menopause helps to normalize it. At the same time as the purification takes place, my body has become the altar housing the light that wants to shine. I believe that a healthy balance of the female and male energies needs to be achieved for humanity, justice, peace and joy for everyone. For those of us who believe (in whatever...), let the Goddesses bloom out to their fullest and shine on!

12 The Return of the Pack

Pamela Windle

I was trembling, disoriented, confused; the temperature outside was −20°C (or so it seemed), with ice-cold winds blowing a gale from the north, weaving its way through Derby train station as I stood there shaking and unable to move.

I was frozen, in fear.

What had just happened? What was I going to do now? How was I going to pay my bills and buy food? How was I going to live? And oh my god, will I get better? I had fatigue that wouldn't go away, doctors couldn't tell me why or show me how to get better, and it was likely to worsen. Those were a few of the thoughts that went through my mind.

The reassuring voice on the end of the phone said, 'Everything is going to be okay; you'll be fine – get home and get warm.'

That was February 7th, 2014. You see, I remember it like it was yesterday. I was being pushed out of full-time employment on capabilities with the equivalent of two months' salary in the bank, and I was ill. Today, when I think about the whole ordeal, I remember how stressful, frightening, physically and emotionally painful, how overwhelming it was. Trying to prove to my boss, who I considered a friend, that what I was going through wasn't fake news felt like a betrayal of our friendship at a time when I was being betrayed by my body.

I decided to leave my employment before I was pushed, which was recommended by my union rep, so I had the dreaded conversation with my boss. I walked out of her office with my head down, to not make eye contact with anyone just in case they saw it – fear. 'Goodbye everyone,' I said in a high-pitched voice, trying to be cheerful and not give anything away as I put my coat and scarf on and my handbag on my shoulder. 'See you soon,' I said, knowing that I wouldn't see them again. Some barely noticed that I was leaving, not even raising their heads from the computer screen as they were drowning in case notes; others smiled and said, 'Yep, bye, see ya.' 'When are you back to work?' 'I'm not sure,' I said, turning away and starting the long walk down the corridor. That day it felt longer than normal.

I held it all in and thought I had gotten away with it until one of my colleagues caught me as I was about to walk out of the door for the last time. 'What's wrong, where are you going?' she said. 'I can't say, but I won't be coming back.' We did all we could to fight back the tears. We hugged. That was it.

The rest is history, so they say, but how did I reclaim 'my six-pack', my health and ultimately my joy?

Slow, slow, very slow

Let's start with the end in mind. In 2018, I sat down in my GP surgery and nervously said, 'I'd like you to amend my medical records to say that I no longer have chronic fatigue syndrome' (CFS, or CFS/ME, is a condition that causes extreme tiredness and a range of other symptoms, such as taking a long time to recover from physical activities, problems with memory, etc.). Phew, I had said it, I had said those words out loud – 'I no longer have chronic fatigue syndrome.' Oh my god, what will she think? My inner voice was on high alert.

She appeared to be slightly hesitant at my request at first, and then nodded and asked, 'Tell me about your CFS, and what did you do to get better?' In my head, I thought to myself, 'Oh boy, I don't think you're going to take me seriously when I tell you how I healed my body after being house-bound for five years.'

So, the story goes like this. One morning, in October 2012, I woke up completely drenched in sweat and with a banging headache; I could barely make it downstairs to get some paracetamol, make myself a cup of Lemsip and get a hot water bottle.

The newly made bedsheets were welcoming, but as I placed the hot Lemsip on the bedside glass table, the mug slipped out of my hand, and hot Lemsip flowed out all over my newly made bedsheet. 'Oh f***!' I felt so weak that I didn't have the energy to remake the bed, so I lay on the opposite side. That was enough for a sick woman. I was done; I was able to give in.

I had the flu. But what's the big deal with that? Everyone gets the flu at some point, don't they? You expect to get better with some 'RnR'.

March 2013 was when I was finally able to work full-time hours. At that point, I thought I had finally recovered. The GP had run various tests, such as white and red blood markers, cortisol levels and hormones FSH (follicle-stimulating hormone) and LH (luteinizing hormone). He likened the results of my hormones to a Lamborghini and not a Morris Minor. 'Not bad for a 46-year-old', he said, happily grinning to himself. For the life of me, I don't remember what my FSH and LH levels were, and if I did, to be quite honest, I didn't have a clue what it meant at that time, but what he said sounded positive.

During that year, I had weeks where I didn't feel myself. I couldn't put my finger on what or how I felt; it was odd. My whole body, brain, arms and legs were as if I was submerged in a sea of thick, sticky treacle. Slow, very slow. Everything was slow, my brain and movements, and my throat hurt so bad it was painful to speak. I couldn't bear daylight at times, and I couldn't sit upright for long periods. I soon developed a habit of slouching or leaning back to avoid using more energy.

The name is Lampshade

I was proud of my six-pack. As a certified personal trainer, I'd consider myself an athlete – well, I was as fit and as strong as one, and I was able to do 65 press-ups in one minute, squat 40kg, and lift my body weight. I ran a few half marathons, taught fitness classes such as Body Pump, Spin and Aqua

Aerobics, and I had auditioned for the Gladiators once! That was an experience. I was going to be called 'Lampshade'... hahaha. I was a fitness junky. My body was a temple, and it still is today, even more so, but differently, and I'll tell you more about that later.

But I had to stop. I had no choice. I stopped for a week, and then I was back at work, living my life the way I did, going to the gym after work, driving up the M1 to Leeds to see my daughter at university, spending time with my new then-partner, visiting family members and socializing. You know, the normal stuff. Slow, stop and repeat – and then it would happen all over again. I had a recurring sore throat and weakness; I couldn't think clearly, I couldn't cope with the demands of work, and it wasn't long before 'they' wanted me out!

It was Notting Hill Carnival, and, oh boy, would I have driven us 127 miles down the M1 and back home that August Bank Holiday if I knew what I know now? Probably. Well, that was the last day I drove any distance for the next five years. Slow, stop and stuck.

That was it. I was house-bound for five years. I felt be-trayed by my friends, GP and my body. Some said, 'It's not going to get any better, and you'll most likely develop fibro-myalgia'; 'You don't look like you have CFS'; 'I have a friend who has that, you need to get back to work'... (Well, I would have if I could have.) 'I can prescribe you an antidepressant.' But was I depressed, I thought to myself? A big fat 'NO' was the voice inside my head. I politely declined her offer, 'It will make you feel better,' she said. 'No thank you.' She didn't have to mutter a word; her body language said it all

– well, suit yourself. And I am glad I did! Don't get me wrong, there were dark times in those long, frightening five years. I remember rummaging through my kitchen cupboard, desperately searching for paracetamol to end it all, researching Google for pain-free ways to die by suicide, and at that point, I reached out for help; encouraged by my partner, I went for counselling.

The healing journey

A new online friend popped a message into my inbox. It read like this: 'Thought this might be of interest to you. Join this Facebook Group called 3rd Age Women. There are other health and wellness pros in there; you'll love it.' It wasn't long before I had enrolled on the 3rd Age Women practitioner online course. I was keen to learn about perimenopause and menopause for myself, mostly because my eldest sister started having hot flushes while organizing our dad's funeral in June 2014.

All I knew about menopause was the misinformation that you grow old and fat, are no longer desirable, dry, and have hot sweats. Seeing my sister, who's four years older than me, sweating like that, for no reason, or so it seemed, left me wanting to know more about this dreaded thing called 'menopause'.

I passed! Yay! The course was fantastic; I learned so much about the female body in this phase of life, how it's possible to slow down the ageing process, support bone and heart health, pelvic floor health, and so much more, and I was hungry for more knowledge. The women I was working with were getting better, their sleep had improved, they were starting to lose weight, their hot flushes decreased, and yet I was still struggling with extreme fatigue, brain fog (now I had a name for it) and muscle stiffness.

A year later, I met Dr Jessica Drummond who had flown in from the USA at a women's health conference in London – she is the founder and CEO of the Integrative Women's Health Institute.[1] I was already on her mailing list and aware of her certified Women's Health Coach year-long qualification, but it was way out of my price range. Being desperate to learn more, something inside me was saying 'you need to do this', so I took the opportunity to meet her.

The course was 5k, which was 50 per cent of the money I had left in my bank account after selling my house and living on my equity for two years. I was haemorrhaging money, with very little coming in even though I had cut my cloth to reduce spending. With limited energy to work and earn a living, and no support from our government, the stream was running dry.

This was a major risk, but I signed up and decided to pay over several months rather than all in one go, even though it would have been cheaper. I hit 'Pay'! Gulp, I've done it. I'm committed to this now. I hadn't told a soul. My email pinged; it read: 'Congratulations, here's your confirmation of purchase, the course start date is May 5th, 2016.' My eyes bulged out of my head as I couldn't believe what I was seeing – it could have been any other date, but it was two years to the day of my dad's passing. I knew it was a sign!

---

1   https://integrativewomenshealthinstitute.com

Dr Jessica offered all students a complementary health coaching call, so, of course, I was going to take advantage of that; I'd be stupid not to. It was a call like I'd never had before. I felt at ease, understood and heard. I left the call feeling like there was finally hope.

My treatment plan

We ran a few diagnostic tests. I'd never heard of any of these beforehand. They were the DUTCH Complete™ (24-hour hormonal test), Organic Acids Test (immune, gut health and nutrition deficiency test) and GI EcologiX™ (gut microbiome test), and I waited nervously for the results. I was so glad that I had Dr Jessica's expertise to help me interpret the results; the information was extremely comprehensive.

I felt as if I was finally able to breathe. Having someone alongside to support me was certainly worth every pound. So now we had a plan. The plan entailed adding herbs such as parsley and coriander and spices such as cinnamon, nutmeg, honey and liquorice root, and cutting out many plant-based foods such as certain legumes, many spices, nuts and seeds, and green leafy vegetables. It was a low oxalate diet, which is considered to be therapeutic and temporary while the gut heals. Oxalate is a by-product of all plant-based foods, with some foods higher in oxalates than others, such as spinach, garlic, onion and black pepper. High oxalate levels can interfere with iron absorption and increase the risk of breast cancer.

Ah, I also forgot to tell you that I had a recurring low iron status – well, ferritin levels; at the lowest, it was 3mcg/dL, which explained why my hair was falling out. Over many years I had many extensive and invasive tests and scans at the hospital, which all were inconclusive. The low-oxalate diet worked!

So, my hormones and adrenal glands were in the peri-menopause phase but not depleted (thank goodness); I was detoxifying oestrogen well, mostly; this is called methylation, and the stool test showed that my immune system was struggling. 'Was this a clue as to why I had CFS?' I wondered. It was.

We decided to run one other test, Epstein-Barr. Bingo! That was it. Epstein-Barr virus belongs to the same family as glandular fever. Even though I no longer had the virus, I had elevated antibodies that caused my body to act as if I had an active virus.

The next step was to starve the virus as it lives in the gut, so we switched everything on its head, and instead of eating only meat as a source of protein, I temporarily ate plant-based protein and a heap of antimicrobial foods such as oregano, thyme, ginger, pepper, lemongrass, basil, onion and garlic (at last, mmmm, flavour – it had been five months). I also had green cabbage, broccoli, Brussels sprouts, kale, red apples, kohlrabi, lemon, lime, green tea and dandelion, to name just a few, as well as targeted supplements including Optimal Liposomal Glutathione, Holy basil, L-lysine, selenium, CoQ10 and CBD oil.

The healing began

My energy levels started to increase incrementally, the

bloating disappeared, and I could think clearly. 'Oh, my joy is returning! I almost feel like the old me.' These words are engraved on my mind. Dr Jessica said, 'We need to get your energy levels up before you reach menopause!' I was 53, which was the first time I skipped a cycle (39 days instead of my usual 26 days).

What's it all got to do with menopause? Everything.

Hand on heart, I can honestly say that if I hadn't been unwell and found a way to heal my body, I would be like so many other women who come to see me in my clinic, struggling with the debilitating hormonal symptoms as they transition into the menopause and beyond. The list is endless: brain fog, energy issues, painful joints, sleep issues, low libido, uncontrollable hot flushes, stubborn weight loss, and so on.

I have had terrible night sweats and hot flushes, which coincided with my mum passing away as we watched over her bedside for three days and nights in January 2020. It took me some time to realize that the stress of mum passing had triggered a cortisol response, hence why my bed was drenched and my face was streaming with sweat... My partner was thoughtful when I was sweating, probably because he's learned about the whole-body approach to menopause subliminally.

There are estimated to be over 50 different hormones in the body, and they all work together, and when one hormone is down, so are the others. It's like a stack of dominoes. Those hormones are also interconnected to the body systems – the digestive system, the endocrine system, the skeletal system, the nervous system, detoxification pathways and neurotransmitters in the brain – and by the time we get to our 40s, 50s and 60s, our bodies have been through a lot – relationship breakdowns, grief, empty nest syndrome, certain medications like the pill, antibiotics, illness, life stressors, and, not forgetting the elephant in the room, the racial prejudice and discrimination from the day I left my mother's care and right through life, including entering into the education system.

To thrive through the perimenopause into menopause and beyond, we must put our needs first, take a whole-body approach and stop thinking that there's one magic pill, supplement or food that will elevate our symptoms. That's simply clever marketing. To date, I have used my experience to help hundreds of perimenopausal, menopausal and postmenopausal women regain their lost energy, sleep throughout the night, wake up feeling energized, increase their libido, lift their mood, lose stubborn weight gain, overcome relationship breakdowns, increase their confidence, and feel like themselves again by resetting their hormones.

As I write this chapter, I'm approaching my 56th birthday, and it's now 183 days since my last bleed, so I'm guessing that I'm almost at the end of perimenopause and about to enter menopause. Mum was in her late 50s too. Genetics plays a huge role, and as I slowly move into being a crony, I honour my body much deeper; she is a temple. Indeed, I love myself more than ever, and am proud of who I've become. I have my six-pack back! ;-) I am healed.

13 The Invisible Cracks

Myrle Roach

There was an age in my life's journey when I felt completely indomitable. The world was mine to do with as I pleased, and nothing, absolutely nothing, could defeat me. As a young Black woman, I felt a certain arrogant pride in the saying 'Black don't crack', knowing that I was guaranteed decades of being 'young' way beyond any standard expiry date given to others whose genetics lack the priceless pigment of melanin. At that stage, monthly confirmations of my womanhood were viewed more as a regular nuisance interrupting the smooth running of my otherwise pain-free life. Monthly cycles and their ebb and flow were not subjects for intense discussion, and I became adept at handling PMS (premenstrual syndrome) and cramps, and with no understanding of the implications, I looked forward to the time when I could put this all behind me. Wondering why it wasn't called 'meno-end', I had no idea of the complexities that came with pressing 'pause' on menstruation.

Explanations on the female rite of passage into woman-hood did not come with intimate chats sharing insights into the meaning of becoming a woman while discovering the answers to searching questions. So, looking further ahead to the end of that journey and the start of a new one was shrouded in mystery, and, to some of us, even more taboo. This was most likely because the women we looked to had never experienced what we looked to them for, so could not fulfil our needs. They equipped us with the logistic know-ledge of what was needed for our monthly validation with stern warnings of repercussions and consequences if you played the 'big woman' now. What we had no idea of was that these strong women were themselves beginning to deal with changes in their bodies that they had not been prepared for, and which had literally ambushed them. We, the daughters, were left to come to terms with the various complexities of menstruation while they began to navigate the minefield of menopause. Thus continues a cycle of fortitude, presenting a façade of stoicism to the world while covering the cracks beneath the surface.

Menstruation and puberty brought for me a new body and a new curiosity about my anatomy and that restricted area of my own body that I had absolutely no idea what it looked like. Suddenly, it became the focal point of my thoughts, and not because it seemed to bleed of its own free will once a month, which apparently was the penalty I paid for being born female and now growing into womanhood. This point hidden between my two legs seemed to come to life on its own and was starting to create sensations that started deep within my belly, radiating outwards. I had never encountered those feelings before and had no idea how to satisfy the strange urges that seemed connected to my blossoming breasts and their throbbing nipples. What was going on? My mind was a jigsaw of questions that needed connecting, but the pieces would not fit where I put them in my head. My teenage years became a maze through which I tried to navigate with no older sister to turn to for answers. At 15, I lost my dad to whom I had always felt closer than I did to my sternly religious mother, who herself had lost the love of her life. We were both grieving, but doing it in solitude. And at the same time, my body had suddenly become an intriguing alien that I wanted to explore while being acutely aware of the inbred restrictions of this taboo activity.

On the surface, I was a thriving teenager, blossoming into an attractive young lady who, when she looked in the mirror, liked what she saw, despite being what was termed a 'big-boned girl'. And it soon became apparent that the young males also found her attractive, and the kiss–chase games became more exploratory and intense. However, the questions going around and around in my head did not receive any answers, and so the first cracks beneath the surface began to appear. I now realized that the taboo subject of 'sex' was occupying my thoughts more and more, and that the forbidden was beckoning to me with promises of pleasure unknown and to be enjoyed. The dots were connecting, but, like the small print on a contract, the real 'facts of life' were not readily available and would only become known through the voyage of experience. The navigation process became mixed with turbulence, instability and some chaos. The world saw the perfect picture of a blossoming 'strong Black woman' whose beauty had a warranty that would not expire because 'Black don't crack'.

The myth of the strength of the Black woman became the trademark that the world expected to see in myself and my ebony, cocoa, caramel and mocha sisters. This came from different areas of society, including our own communities. We carry a heavy legacy from slavery of being labelled as childbearing machines that allow us to produce with a lack of emotion while labouring in the fields and great houses, pausing to deliver, and then continuing to toil. This fabrication has put us Black women at a disadvantage for centuries, making us and our health needs one of the most misunderstood of the female species. Our bodies have long been viewed as machines that don't need maintenance and preservation or to be treated with care and understanding. So, when we approach medical professionals for their support, guidance and treatment, is it any wonder that many of us are dismissed with a lack of effort to fully comprehend our problems? The fact that overall women's bodies have always been presented as an enigma to the male-dominated medical profession makes the Black woman's case even more difficult to resolve. Many of us are taken at face value with no attempt to look beyond the surface and see the cracks.

I went through pregnancy and childbearing, once again unprepared for another female rite of passage – giving birth. But being the 'strong Black woman' I was supposed to be, my body did what was expected and naturally delivered a beautiful 8lb 9oz baby, which saw me being proud of my childbearing hips and this achievement. So, still not completely accepting that the only guaranteed contraception is abstinence, I was soon pregnant again, this time naturally delivering a 10lb baby, which left me traumatized, and despite my fairy-tale plans for three children, the baby production factory closed. After making this firm decision, I put my trust in 'The Pill', and then my eyes became opened to the full discovery of the joys of sexual pleasure. And as society began to change its views and be more accepting and forthcoming about sexuality, I enjoyed a full and pleasurable time with no inhibitions to giving into the demands of my healthy sex drive. At this point, the word 'perimenopause' did not even exist in my vocabulary, and I enjoyed the freedom of my 30s and 40s, believing that the best was probably yet to come! I was totally unaware of the cracks that were slowly developing below the surface and the impact they would have on my carefree life.

Then, just like that, even though I did not look 50, I completed my half-century and proudly defied the ageist syndrome, reiterating that 'Black don't crack'. But then the warning signals began to make an appearance camouflaged as prevalent health issues in the Black community. I went from always having a good blood pressure reading of 110/60 mmHg to a sky-high reading of 140/90 mmHg, resulting in being attached to a machine that pumped up and beeped every hour on the hour to record my pressure. No surprise that my male doctor was completely baffled as to what was causing the ongoing headaches and high blood pressure. Being a 'strong Black woman', I didn't see the need to mention mood swings and insomnia because I just thought the headaches were making me irritable. When my sex drive began to diminish, I blamed it on the headaches too, and didn't need to fabricate an excuse to avoid intimacy. Having switched to a coil a few years before as my failsafe method of contraception, irregular menstrual periods were not a concern. Nothing made me even consider that my body was transitioning into menopause. It took a problem with my coil and a visit with a female medical practitioner who specialized in contraception, leading to a subsequent blood test, to be eventually told that I was going through perimenopause.

The focus of the lady seated in front of me was to discuss the pros and cons of removing the current wandering coil and whether I should have another one inserted. Glancing at the file in front of her with my information, I saw her pause, focus on something written on the page in front of her and then look at me. Then she said, 'I didn't realize you are 50!' To which I flippantly replied, 'Nearly 51.' The conversation that ensued left me even more confused and I departed her office with the word 'perimenopause' ringing in my ears. This was the very first time that I had heard the word. My simplified understanding of my reproductive life span was that it started with menstruation and ended with menopause. What the hell was perimenopause, and what was happening to my body because of it? Was this another subject shrouded in mystery and restrictions that women were supposed to figure out all on their own?

I was then referred to my GP, who, apparently, would clarify everything. This was according to the female medical practitioner after realizing she was younger than me and had no information to give me on a topic that she had no knowledge or personal experience of. Her discomfort in discussing the topic was obvious as her confident demeanour changed on reading the results of my blood test, and she could not wait to get me out of her office. Once again, my uncrackable surface had caused misguided assumptions about my age and I was sent adrift to another destination for answers. Before going for my appointment with my GP, I threw out the word to a few female friends who were just as bewildered as I was, knowing the 'meno' word but having no idea what adding 'peri' to it meant.

So, I approached my appointment with apprehension, expecting to hear about a possible abnormality or functional defect brought on by my indulgent sex life and implanting foreign bodies to accommodate it. However, my male GP was even more uncomfortable than his female colleague, and somehow made me feel that because I didn't look my age, I was to blame for him never even considering that I was old enough to have started perimenopause, much less to be approaching the end of it. He made short work of explaining anything by sending me on my way with a folded piece of A4 paper to read that should give me the answers I sought. How dare he decide that he knew the answers when he never bothered to find out the questions? And there were so many questions revolving in my head. I now understood the reason for my headaches, high blood pressure, insomnia and other symptoms that had pushed through the cracks. But I had other questions that needed answers, and wondered if this had been brought on by my own actions.

My punishment for living a robust sexual life began as my sex drive went on its downward spiral into non-existence. Unable to explain what I was going through, I found it easier to distance myself even more from my already long-distance lover, and sever what were already tenuous ties. I convinced myself that I was to blame for what was happening to my body, and that the implanted coil, which eventually needed minor surgery to be removed, was the cause. I regarded perimenopause as the punishment for my sins, the ones that I now had absolutely no desire for and didn't miss. Once again, my body had been taken over by an unknown entity that would not synchronize with my brain and, despite the chaos in my head, was not represented on the surface of my existence. Beneath the surface, a myriad of cracks were now rampant and wreaking havoc with my physical existence.

My life became a lonely reality presenting a smooth, smiling countenance to the world, still defying the advancement of age as living proof that 'Black don't crack' was fact and not fiction. Beneath the surface, however, physical changes were taking place that were no longer myths but still a mystery. To this day, I have no idea when I went from perimenopause to actual menopause. I became adept at joking about this transitional rite of passage and would refer to any temperature rises as 'tropical moments' as I had no desire to identify with the age-old term 'hot flushes'. Just my way of daring to defy the monster that was on a destructive rampage throughout my body and mind. I continued to publicly flirt and engage with males who I found cosmetically attractive, but I did not feel one spark of chemistry in the hope that my drive would return and that would mean everything was back to normal. But this never went beyond verbal flirtations as my libido was at an all-time low to the point of being absent, and although I displayed my feminine wiles on the surface, underneath I was feeling less and less like a desirable woman.

No one had explained that just as menstruation brought all the benefits of being a female, menopause would take them away. That it would rob me of not only the power to procreate, but also of the desire to engage in the pleasurable act that accompanied it. I would suddenly be able to look at the sexiest specimen of manhood and feel nothing but aesthetic pleasure. If anyone had told me this 20 years before, I would have made a bargain with the Creator to endure the monthly flow in its entirety for as long as possible to allow other juices to keep flowing. I became preoccupied with ensuring that my outward femininity was enhanced and pre-served because beneath the surface it had disappeared, and I was terrified that it would never return. When presenting myself in public, I ensured that I still looked younger than my age and the opposite sex would still express admiration with offers to fulfil my desires, which, unknown to them, were non-existent.

Prior to menstruation, I was a girl enjoying my childhood years and not contemplating anything beyond the next day at school and maybe as far ahead as the next school holidays to run free and uninhibited. The arrival of what I considered to be the monthly curse introduced an entire new world that I fought against at first, but then came to recognize as powers bestowed on me for the honour of being born a female. This elevated me to a different level, and I began my journey through womanhood feeling that these superpowers would immortalize my femininity. I was not prepared in any way for the ambush from menopause, which, to date, has not paused my journey but feels as if it has been brought to a very abrupt end. Even though I have not been plagued by many of the physical symptoms that have bombarded other females, my menopause journey has left me devoid of the essence of what I felt made me a real woman. I now feel a very real emptiness in my core that I am seeking to fill, in the hope that the hidden cracks will be sealed.

Today I continue to smile on the surface while below the façade invisible cracks weep for the woman I once was. They weep for the young girl who tried to understand what was happening to her body but was only warned not to play with boys and never allow anyone to touch her 'there'. Tears stream from those cracks for the teenager who thought that she needed to have sex to prove she was attractive to boys but hated it and then waited a few more years before venturing into that Pandora's box again. The sound of sobs echoes from them for the woman whose body was traumatized by childbirth but so proud of the perfectly formed babies that she delivered. The cracks widened to allow the passing of carefree years of undiluted sexual pleasure that would come to a sudden unexplained ending which is now mourned. How can I warn my younger sisters of a different middle passage that may take them from Motherland to Neverland? How can I prepare them for the invisible cracks and what they bring?

My hope is that committing my story to paper will help uncover some of the mystery that has kept the facts of menopause hidden from generations of Black women, leaving us to meander our lonely way through a maze of myths and half-truths. No longer should the younger generation be left adrift in the storm to navigate without a compass, trying to find the welcome beam of a lighthouse beckoning to a safe harbour. The time has come for Black women of every age to be able to enjoy and be proud of their outer beauty while being armed with the knowledge that although they aren't visible, the cracks will come, and how to be ready for them as they begin to make their presence felt beneath the surface. As we dispel the myths of menopause, we allow all Black women to retain the magic of our melanin. Our stories are ours to tell, and it is time for the world to listen as we share them.

14 Living My Best Life

The Gynaecologist
Dr Leslie Anne Bishop

'Can you have another baby, pleeeease?!'

My younger son had just learned in school that at the menopause, women can no longer have babies, that it typically occurs at age 50, and I was 49!! I had long decided he would be my last child, but there are many women who have not made that decision by the time the menopause comes around. They read in the newspaper that Naomi Campbell had her first baby at age 50 and believe they can, too, while not considering that fertility is significantly reduced at that time, and in-vitro fertilization and surrogacy costs are prohibitive for most.

This can be difficult for high-achieving women who are otherwise 'successful', having built their careers and their homes on their own, and thinking that now the time is right to have a baby. But the ovaries are saying the time is wrong. The proverbial biological clock has stopped ticking and they then go from doctor to doctor, clinic to clinic, trying to get pregnant. I have heard many whisper, with sadness and regret, about the baby they chose not to have when they were 22 years old battling with college and two jobs, and how they wished they had listened to the grandmother who kept asking them when they would have the baby. The grandmother who did not understand why having a career and home would be the priority, and who pointed out the other women in the family, her school friends, the pretty girl down the road, who were on to their second or third child. That same grandmother who was excited to see the new house, but in the same sentence asked about the baby for the other bedroom.

Too many Black women feel pressured to have babies, with their self-worth linked to childbearing, perhaps more than childrearing. How often have we heard that we are not a 'real woman, if you've not had a baby', and that 'men are not interested in brains'? At age 34, 10 years post-graduation, and now with my first son, I was told 'you're finally a real woman'. It's no wonder that many see the menopause as the last chance, believing that 'without a child, I'm a failure'. In the African diaspora, this self-judgement is part of our living history of slavery, and it is accompanied by other negative stereotyping such as our hips are big because they are better for giving birth – not true – and that we have big breasts for breastfeeding.

Modern reproductive healthcare has underpinned this dilemma for women. Reliable, safe contraception has allowed us to delay giving birth until we are ready so that we can maximize our potential in so many aspects of our lives. We can be the dependable aunt, niece or daughter who is always available to help the extended family, but without a child of her own, many Black women feel lonely at menopause. At this phase of their lives, many women are also taking care of their own mothers and they begin to question, 'Who will take care of me, who can I depend on, beyond the menopause, in those "golden years"?' Perhaps adoption is a solution.

'I'm free!! I don't have to worry about getting pregnant again!'

This is the flip-side of arriving at the menopause, at the end of fertility. I celebrated that I can be intimate without the 'crisis' of forgetting to take the pill and no longer needing to consider the numerous side effects of various contraceptive methods.

Our Caribbean men often refuse vasectomies, and long-term contraception inevitably becomes our responsibility. So finally, at the menopause, we can now be spontaneous, and like men, feel the 'world is our oyster'! But even though women at the menopause do not need to use condoms for contraception, they protect us against sexually transmitted diseases. In old and new relationships, if we, or our partners, have other partners, we should negotiate continuing to use condoms. I know that this is not always easy, especially in marriages, as it implies confronting infidelity or 'open' relationships, which we may not want, know how to do or have the courage to deal with. There is also the 'empty nest' situation that gets into relationships and the bedroom because we are no longer 'busy' with the family and children, and when we would have stayed for the children, the children are now gone, so we question – do we stay for ourselves and use condoms, or do we stay, like our mothers and grandmothers did themselves, and told us that we should do, ignoring the risk of STDs (sexually transmitted diseases)? Or do we stay but resolve to use the 'I'm too old for that [sex]' excuse?

'It hurts and I don't feel for it!'

Sex is complicated! Libido is multifactorial in women (and in men, too), and now that we don't have to worry about getting pregnant, our sex drive can be very low. Our ovaries have stopped producing eggs, which is good, but they have also stopped producing oestrogen and testosterone too! We fake it, we discuss it with our friends, with our gynaecologist, and, finally, with our partner. Actually, our partner brings it up with us! 'It's a hormonal thing,' we explain in one sentence, but how do we explain that 'we love you dearly, but just don't want to have sex with you' or anyone else? We feel tired and want to sleep. We are not getting aroused any more, even when we try. The natural lubrication is less, and we struggle with the many homophobic myths around the use of lubricating jelly. We feel bruised and get recurrent bladder symptoms; we take antibiotics, and then get recurrent yeast infections with vulval itching. We know that, if available, we can use a vaginal oestrogen cream, but we feel that 'it's not worth the effort'!

'It takes two to tango!' Many women complain that their partners are older, with medical conditions that affect their performance in the bedroom, and we have seen that the COVID-19 pandemic has brought into full focus that Black people have a higher incidence of co-morbidities, hypertension and diabetes, which are invariably uncontrolled. So even though our men may not admit it, their less firm anatomy, combined with our reduced lubrication, makes dyspareunia (painful intercourse) worse. But it has been instilled in us to respect our Black men's egos, so we end up taking full responsibility rather than persuading our men to seek medical attention. We discuss it with our gynaecologist, but persevere with half the solution, and eventually we give up on that aspect of our lives, often much sooner than we really want to!

'I have to pee every minute!'

Gone are the days when I would go all day without going to the toilet or of sticking to my vow never to use a toilet outside of my home. 'Typically, I can hold it until reaching the front door, then I must go straight to the toilet because the pee starts running down my legs before I can get my underwear off!' This is a usual description of urgent urinary incontinence due to the loss of oestrogen, which occurs with the climacteric (encompassing perimenopause, menopause and postmenopause) affecting the bladder and urethra too. The bladder leaking urine during the day may require the use of panty shields, even when not menstruating, and some women complain of self-awareness of an odour, not detected by anyone else, but causing avoidance of social interaction. There may be sensation of a 'lump coming down' in the vagina, which is worse with coughing or a bowel movement, and this uterovaginal prolapse may be confirmed by clinical exam by a gynaecologist. Unfortunately, many of us do not seek medical attention for these symptoms because we believe that they are a 'normal' part of ageing, or because of the social stigma of the genitourinary syndrome of the menopause, or GSM.[1]

What is helpful is reducing the risk factors such as obesity, diabetes, constipation and chronic cough, and, in mild cases, the first line of treatment is pelvic floor muscle exercises such as Kegel exercises. Bladder retraining can also be done by going to the toilet by the clock, initially every two hours, then increasing by half an hour every week, until voluntarily going every three to four hours, with no leaks in between.

As a gynaecologist, I suggest that the exercises are done in 10 repetitions, three times a day for three months, and apart from reducing urinary incontinence and prolapse, the exercises tighten the vaginal muscle walls, which can lead to increased sexual pleasure during intercourse.

'I don't want to have a hysterectomy...'

The climacteric, with the bleeding symptoms of the approaching menopause, may trigger the need for a hysterectomy. Irregular periods, flooding, large clots, soiled bed linen and embarrassment are usually what prompts us to seek a drastic solution. You may have heard of the lady in the Bible who had the prolonged periods for 12 years, and in desperation broke all the purity laws of the day, to touch the clothes of Jesus and be cured (Mark 5:25–34)!

---

1   Kim, H. K., Kang, S. Y., Chung, Y. J., Kim, J. H. and Kim, M. R. (2015) 'The recent review of the genitourinary syndrome of menopause.' *Journal of Menopausal Medicine* 21(2), 65–71. https://doi.org/10.6118/jmm.2015.21.2.65

Unfortunately, some women experience the menopause cold turkey, meaning that their functional ovaries have been removed surgically, often for health reasons. This causes their oestrogen hormone level to drop off suddenly, unlike the gradual fall-off that happens with the naturally occurring menopause. The hot flashes, night sweats and mood changes can sometimes happen even before discharge from hospital. This type of surgical menopause that I had was easier because I had anticipated the symptoms, and they were acknowledged by the caregivers, and myself. But even without the physical symptoms, the emotions associated with the loss of the womb, the loss of my Black womanhood, cannot be ignored.

Having a hysterectomy is a major decision. And like all major decisions, it should be well thought through, the risks and benefits discussed and all options explored. Unfortunately, Black women, with a significantly higher incidence of symptomatic uterine fibroids, are faced with this decision more often than other groups. Our mothers and grandmothers probably faced the same decision, too. Thankfully, modern alternatives, such as uterine artery embolization, are available and are ideal for some women. In the past, the patriarchal approach to healthcare meant that our mothers were perhaps not informed or involved in determining which intervention was best suited to them.

There are, however, some conditions, such as some gynaecological cancers, that do require treatment by hysterectomy, and in those settings, delaying surgery because of ignorance, or fear of the menopause, is not a safe option and can result in the need for more extensive surgery and a worse outcome.

It is not always that our ovaries need to be removed at

the time of the hysterectomy – it depends on the underlying problem – so sometimes the womb is removed and the ovaries conserved. Although that will be the end of periods, and the associated bleeding problems, surgery will have less impact on our hormones, and symptoms may be due to our ovaries producing less and less oestrogen. Removing them at the time of the hysterectomy mimics the natural menopause. Removing ovaries and shutting off our oestrogen may at times be necessary to prevent breast cancer in high-risk women, or part of a treatment protocol for those already diagnosed with the condition. Surgery, knowledge and support in these scenarios is the answer.

'Can't get rid of this fat tummy!'

Central to our sense of our sex appeal is our self-image, and for many of us, self-image is not only determined by self or what we see in the mirror, but also by what our friends, family, culture, their culture, tell us. Multiple factors contribute to the 'fat tummy' that won't budge. I am told, and photos confirm, that I had a 'flat tummy' in my 20s. At 40-plus, my on-and-off battle with the bulge began. Diet and exercise worked! At 50+ it was harder, and I could partially blame the onset of the menopause and the hormonal changes for the central obesity. Harder to exercise for a minimum of 30 minutes a day, five days a week. Harder to be disciplined with my diet – reduce empty sweet calories, drink hot green tea and ice-cold water. I knew that ice cream reduced my stress, as did 'just one block' of dark chocolate! I also knew that pounding the treadmill made me feel better. Stress-related binge-eating released endorphins, and so did exercise.

There is a recognized increase in subcutaneous fat, which we see in the mirror, and visceral fat, which surrounds our internal organs.[2] This 'fat tummy' is associated with increased risk of insulin resistance and type 2 diabetes, already more prevalent in the Black community, and the COVID-19 pandemic has identified worse outcomes in diabetes, which is known to increase the chances of heart disease. With diabetes in pregnancy, and a strong family history, my own risk was increased.

So, it's more than my sex appeal. I persevere, watching my diet and exercise, reducing stress and 'knowing my numbers' – body weight, waist circumference, blood pressure, blood sugar and cholesterol levels.

'I never remember where I've put my keys!'

Not sure if this started when I was perimenopausal, but I certainly recall spending 10 minutes every morning looking for the car or house keys. Being a 'list person' saved me – writing my 'to-do list' every night in a small diary that fit in my handbag. Of course, some items remained undone from one day to the next, but structure masked this underlying climacteric symptom that my friends spoke about. Eventually,

2   de Mutsert, R., Gast, K., Widya, R., de Koning, E., Jazet, I., Lamb, H., le Cessie, S., de Roos, A., Smit, J., Rosendaal, F. and den Heijer, M. (2018) 'Associations of abdominal subcutaneous and visceral fat with insulin resistance and secretion differ between men and women: The Netherlands Epidemiology of Obesity Study.' *Metabolic Syndrome and Related Disorders* 16(1), 54–63.

I got a basket to put my keys in at night! I had to make a shopping list for the supermarket, too, or I would return every day, making unnecessary holes in my finances.

We have known that a fall in oestrogen levels at menopause is linked with memory loss, and recent studies suggest that it is also linked to the long-standing racism to which Black women are exposed. It is postulated that racism is a recurrent psychological stress that impacts on cognitive function, including memory, as we get older.[3]

My mother has been doing daily crosswords from the newspaper since in her 50s, to stave off dementia, and she saw her mother do the same. It must be said that there is a difference between 'brain fog' and early dementia – the former is treatable but is now complicated by symptoms of Long COVID. It helps to ensure that I am hearing well and seeing well. If I was running the household, doing a full-time job, taking care of elderly parents and keeping an eye on adult children, I would expect the occasional memory loss that is typical of getting older, like grey hair!

'Is it hot, or is it me?!'

I never experienced hot flashes, although it affects up to 80 per cent of women. Although I had a surgical menopause, my ovaries had probably been slowly producing less oestrogen long before, and I lived by the Caribbean Sea, with cool sea breezes all the time!

---

3   Coogan, P., Schon, K., Li, S., Cozier, Y., Bethea, T. and Rosenberg, L. (2020) 'Experiences of racism and subjective cognitive function in African American women.' *Alzheimer's & Dementia: Diagnosis, Assessment & Disease Monitoring* 12(1).

Hot flashes may last for up to 10 years, but typically up to four years after the menopause. The Women's Health Initiative study initially suggested that hormone replacement therapy (HRT) was too risky to be used for hot flashes, but reanalysis concluded that it was safe in most women under the age of 60.[4] The longitudinal SWAN study noted that Black women were more likely to experience hot flashes, and the symptoms were more severe and lasted for longer, compared with white women. However, they were less likely to take HRT medication.[5] There is evidence that HRT may trigger the growth of uterine fibroids. As Black women have a higher incidence of fibroids, we would require closer monitoring when using HRT.[6]

In Jamaica, despite doctors' knowledge of the efficacy of HRT for menopausal symptoms, they are less likely to prescribe it.[7] In Trinidad and Tobago, women try herbal medicine, exercise or diversion programmes to deal with

---

4 Sood, R., Faubion, S. S., Kuhle, C. L., Thielen, J. M. and Shuster, L. T. (2014) 'Prescribing menopausal hormone therapy: An evidence-based approach.' *International Journal of Women's Health 6*, 47–57. Available at: www.ncbi.nlm.nih.gov/pmc/articles/PMC3897322, accessed 15 February 2022.

5 Harlow, S., Burnett-Bowie, S., Greendale, G., Avis, N., Reeves, A., Richards, T. and Lewis, T. (2022) 'Disparities in reproductive aging and midlife health between black and white women: The Study of Women's Health Across the Nation (SWAN).' *Women's Midlife Health 8*(1).

6 Moro, E., Degli Esposti, E., Borghese, G., Manzara, F., Zanello, M., Raimondo, D., Gava, G., Arena, A., Casadio, P., Meriggiola, M. C. and Seracchioli, R. (2019) 'The impact of hormonal replacement treatment in postmenopausal women with uterine fibroids: A state-of-the-art review of the literature.' *Medicina (Kaunas, Lithuania) 55*(9), 549. https://doi.org/10.3390/medicina55090549

7 Harrison, G. M., Medley, N. N., Carroll, K. N., Simms-Stewart, D. A., Wynter, S. H., Fletcher, H. M. and Rattray, C. A. (2021) 'Mind the gap: Primary care physicians and gynecologists' knowledge about menopause and their attitudes to hormone therapy use in Jamaica.' *Menopause 28*(12), 1385–1390. https://doi.org/10.1097/GME.0000000000001854

their symptoms.[8] Some women in Tobago use nutritional supplements containing magnesium, zinc and vitamin D. My informal survey of the pharmacies in Tobago revealed that nearly two-thirds did not have HRT preparations in stock, suggesting the use of alternatives.

Hot flashes may also be an indicator of overactive thyroid disease, which can present at the same time as the menopause. Similarly, the lack of energy or inertia may reflect an underactive thyroid. Both diagnoses can be confirmed with a blood test and treated to relieve the symptoms that mimic the climacteric.

'So, what can we do?'

We have a history of being 'strong Black women', which has often been used against us in addressing our health issues. But we must not give up our strengths, our mentoring, our sisterhood in dealing with the menopause. The symptoms of the menopause are due to the hormonal changes at the penultimate phase of a woman's reproductive life. How many of us can recall puberty, with the pimples and moodiness, when it all started?

The introduction of the combined oral contraceptive pill – the COC – in the 1960s has changed the lives of women, and the world. For the first time, women could safely decide if,

---

8   Elbourne, K.T. (2018) 'Menopausal transition and its association with the quality of life of women aged 40–55 of varying ethnicity in county St Patrick West, Trinidad: A community-based survey.' *Journal of Women's Health Care*. Available at: www. longdom.org/proceedings/menopausal-transition-and-its-association-with-the-quality-of-life-of-women-aged-4055-of-varying-ethnicity-in-county-st--42062.html, accessed 14 February 2022.

when, with whom and how many children to birth, allowing us to traverse our reproductive lives differently from our mothers and grandmothers. It is hoped that the advances in healthcare will continue to help us to control the unpredictable climacteric symptoms and that the COC, in low doses, will continue to be useful for many women up to the menopause, in providing contraception, as well as reducing bleeding, bloating, hot flashes, pelvic pain and the risk of ovarian cancer, for convenient scheduling of periods, and as an alternative to the hysterectomy for non-cancer conditions. HRT, with even lower doses of oestrogen than the COC, can supplement the lack of our natural oestrogens, with reduced risk. Admittedly, there is a small group of women who should not take oestrogen preparations because of the breast cancer risk, VTE (venous thromboembolism, or blood clot) risk or smoking; progesterone-only preparations and non-hormonal therapies are alternatives.

The COVID-19 pandemic has exposed the social disparities that affect Black women with a higher incidence of comorbidities, including obesity. We often try our traditional remedies and sometimes delay accessing modern health options, but it is important for us as a collective to embrace our supportive companionships, the teas and the tips, while also considering the new alternatives.

As a postmenopausal Black woman, I am very self-aware, having survived life's challenges and learned many lessons, so I can share, guide, mentor and still learn some more. I know what works and what doesn't, and what a healthy lifestyle means for me. I have SMART goals and know how much I want to weigh, what I should eat and how I could sometimes cheat my diet! I have a realistic exercise routine, which doesn't happen every day, but often enough to release the endorphins and keep my numbers down.

I choose my relationships, professional and personal, wisely, and I trust my gut. I can truthfully acknowledge the relationships that enrich me, those that do not, and how to manoeuvre the difference. I also know the impact of stress on my physical, mental and emotional health, how to reduce it, avoid it or get help. I know how to be intimate with myself or with others, what gives me pleasure and what doesn't, and I am enjoying it because I want to, not because I feel obliged to.

I am now 10 years post the menopause and living my best life! I've never felt better!

15 My Fluctuating Libido

Tashini Jones

I have often wondered if the lack of conversations about periods and menopause is a generational thing, a cultural reality, or both? I never once heard my Jamaican mother, my aunties or her friends ever mention anything significant around the menstrual cycle except to ask me if I needed pads. When it came to the menopause, I only ever heard the odd thing about hot flushes, and that silence is why I thought that is all it was about. Maybe my mother and aunties were embarrassed to talk to a young girl about those things because they would have then had to go into details about it. But menopause was heading my way, and I was now grown, yet I still could not understand why the conversation never happened. But thinking about it, at no point in my life did I hear any conversations from my mother and aunties about sex or anything else related to physical intimacy. Most of my female friends say that they experienced the same thing, and so I entered my menopause blindly, unprepared for the 'baptism of fire', which was very much an understatement.

I foolishly went through my 20s, 30s and 40s praying for menopause to happen so that my awful periods would go away and stop taking over my life. I would sit and dream of the days where I would no longer have to carry half my wardrobe around in my handbag, and that I could have sex morning, noon and night on tap, without any fears or interruptions. That did not last for long because when the reality of menopause took its grip, I was unprepared for the mental or physical changes and challenges I would face. It was terrifying.

My menopause started in my 40s and I had just come out of a relationship and was very unaware of most of the physical changes happening to my body. I was sexually inactive for several years and, to be honest, I was not missing it – to this day I am not sure if the lack of interest was caused by the menopause, my mental and emotional state or just my personal desire, but either way, it was not on the cards. Let me just say that I was not prepared for the issues I had when I did start a new sexual relationship.

The new relationship began about four or five years into my menopause, and I was looking forward to the physical side of it. I thoroughly enjoyed sex throughout my adulthood, and I am going to get a little bit graphic here, but this is just to emphasize how things were and not to cause any sensationalism.

I remember our first time together. I was eager, ready and more than willing to fully participate in it all. My first stumbling block was my hips. I had developed mild arthritis after the menopause started, and while it had not interrupted most of my daily activities, having my partner bear down on my hips with his full body weight brought a new kind of hip pain I had never encountered. All I could think of at the time was that I wanted this man to get off me so the pain would subside. He then thought of a clever suggestion – let's change position – but for me it was impossible to have penetrative sex without hip involvement, so trying other positions just brought another wave of hip pain that I really could not stand. This pain was a completely new and unpleasant sensation. I had always been overweight before my menopause, yet I never, ever had an issue getting into any position, nor felt pain trying some of those gymnastic Karma Sutra-type positions.

This was a new experience for me. All I can say is that the pain was intense – my body was shaking, and he misread that to think that I was heading toward orgasm. He had a great time, but I felt thoroughly deflated and quite upset that the sex had been so traumatic for me. I ran to the bathroom afterwards, and when I began cleaning myself, I noticed a blood smear that I put down to 'vaginal inactivity'. I did not let it bother me until I noticed it was happening every time we had sex. I was so traumatized by it that I didn't even want oral sex because I was scared that would also trigger the bleeding. I wondered, was the issue his heavy-handedness in my nether regions? Because there are some men who think that the vagina is indestructible and made of reinforced material like concrete or steel, and that they can manhandle it to a ridiculous degree, thinking that the battering is enjoyable, and not painful or uncomfortable. To be honest, the bleeding had me so worried that I took myself off the GP. I did not know the cause and was not taking any chances with my health. I was lucky to be allocated a female doctor that day and did not have a smidgen of embarrassment describing my symptoms to her. She was able to diagnose the issue and described it as a thinning of my vaginal walls caused by the lack of oestrogen. I felt reassured knowing that it was quite common during menopause, She suggested using vaginal moisturizer to help alleviate the pain and the bleeding, and it was then that I found out the difference between a lubricant and vaginal moisturizer. I was glad to have that newfound knowledge because even though I was self-lubricating, as I always have done, I just could not understand the soreness. If you do not know the difference, pause here, Google it, and you can thank me later.

So, with prescription in hand, off I went to the pharmacy to get that much-needed relief, and, for a short while, until the moisturizer started doing its thing, I found every excuse imaginable not to have any kind of sexual encounter. I just could not face the painful physical feelings I had been getting and the toll it was taking on my mental health – the possibility of a sexual encounter presenting itself would cause my anxiety levels to go through the roof.

A couple of months into using the moisturizer, I was watching TV with my 30-year-old goddaughter and an advert about a brand of vaginal moisturizer popped up. She then exclaimed in horror, 'Why would they advertise that on TV?' I rolled my eyes and responded, 'In 20 years from now you won't be asking such a stupid question!' while chuckling to myself and praying I would still be around to remind her of her question. At that time, I also discovered how great CBD creams were for my arthritis because the hip pain was waning, and I felt like I was regaining some kind of control of my body. I was feeling better physically, but my mental health was not playing ball at all.

The relationship was still in its infancy, but with all the aggravation I was going through, I began reflecting, and it dawned on me that maybe the vaginal tightness and the impossibility of pleasurable penetration was my body's way of telling me that I should not be having a sexual relationship with this particular person. I knew that the moisturizer was doing its job and the bleeding had stopped, but now I was being tortured with something else – I could not stop wondering whether the painful penetration was a psychological thing or whether it was only physical. I just could not figure it out, but what I do know is that it got to the point where I did not even want to be touched by him. Because while I was being traumatized during sex, he was finding it wonderful and pleasurable. He described it as his 'dick being grabbed and held tight by my pussy'. His enthusiasm definitely far outstripped mine. Now that I am writing this, I have to giggle, because back in the day, when I was younger, whenever I said size matters, I meant the bigger the better; now when I say size matters, I mean small is great – anything bigger than a Kit Kat chocolate finger biscuit will made me weep with sheer agony.

I did not bother going back to the GP; instead, I consulted 'Dr Google'. I searched the internet, and in less than a minute I found out that it was not my waning desire for this man that made intercourse difficult but that it was a very real physical condition that affects many menopausal women like myself. I found out from 'Dr Google' that vaginal atrophy, or atrophic vaginitis, was the medical name for the symptoms I had been experiencing – dryness, tightness, burning, bleeding and urinary incontinence (there are many more symptoms, and an online search will find them). I was quite taken aback to know that roughly 45 per cent of postmenopausal women experience symptoms of vaginal atrophy[1] – so how come I had not known about this before? Lewis says that we are afraid to mention the words 'vaginal atrophy', but she found the courage to speak out to family and friends about her situation and never felt alone because of this.[2]

I do not know whether vaginal atrophy affects women, femmes, trans and non-binary people more if they have been sexually inactive during their early menopause or not, but what I do know from many conversations I have had is that it seems to affect those who have abstained from sex for prolonged periods of time.

I asked a family member how she managed sex during her menopause and she said, 'It constantly changes – one minute I'm cold and don't want him near me, and next I'm behaving like I'm auditioning for a porn movie.' That pretty much sums it up! Lewis says about the vagina, 'use it or lose it',[3] and I'd like to add that I think the vagina works just like an appliance – which sometimes needs WD40 when it gets rusty – at the very least that definitely describes my vagina to a tee!

1   Goldstein, I., Dicks, B., Kim, N. N. and Hartzell, R. (2021) 'Multidisciplinary overview of vaginal atrophy and associated genitourinary symptoms in postmenopausal women.' *Sexual Medicine* 1(2), 44–53. Available at: www.sciencedirect.com, accessed 12 December 2021.
2   Lewis, J. (2018) *Me & My Menopausal Vagina: Living with Vaginal Atrophy*. PAL Books.
3   Lewis, J. (2018) *Me & My Menopausal Vagina: Living with Vaginal Atrophy*. PAL Books.

I have heard from others who have had severe cases of vaginal atrophy and undergone vaginal rejuvenation or laser therapy surgery. I personally would not have opted for either of those, but one evening, when chatting with friends at varying stages of menopause, one mentioned vaginal dilators – a device that come in sets of various sizes that gently stretches the vagina – starting with the smallest and over time increasing sizes until the vagina feels more natural. I was so sold on the idea that I ordered some online during the middle of our chat, and was so excited that as soon as they arrived, I opened the box and off I went to try them out. I delightfully felt the benefits within a couple of months, and intercourse became less of a painful affair and some of the fear I felt disappeared.

My fluctuating libido took me by surprise, and if my partner so much as looked at me, he would get that side-eye that Black families give to kids when they step out of line. He soon learned the signs and trod carefully. But other times I was like a dog on heat and could not keep my hands off him. It did not make sense to me, and it certainly did not make sense to him, and I know he was resentful. Maybe he felt slighted, especially because of the stereotyping of Black male virility, but there was nothing he could say or do to turn me on, and to be frank, he really ought to consider himself lucky that I even sat in the same room as him because his presence got on my nerves.

I wish I could say I felt guilty about it, but I did not, and I assume that was part of the menopause. I did try to explain the physical changes my body had gone through and was still going through, and that it was never about him personally. I let him know that while he had all the vigour in the world,

I had hit a certain age and my body was changing, so doing adventurous erotic things, like pinning my legs behind my head, no longer worked for me – all it did was cut off my air supply, and something as simple as doggy style was torture because of the arthritis in my knees and hips. I let him know that he had better forget about a quickie in the car because sex in a small space was now Mission Impossible.

I have to be honest and say that during that time I learned a lot about myself and my sexual preferences, because since my menopause so much had changed physically over the years. I learned what stimulates and turns me on, and where once the very sight of a man's naked physique would have me drooling like a St Bernard dog, these days, being treated with love, kindness and compassion is a real turn on for me. Relearning how my vagina works and what it likes and doesn't like, and the ability to speak freely about it, and exploring my body, and the touching of the pleasure spots, have also been very liberating.

Going by my experience, I really do think that it is important to understand the changes we go through and to also relay this to our partners. Thankfully, with modern technology, information can be accessed via websites such as Stanford Health,[4] Web MD[5] and Healthline,[6] and many others. There is a wealth of useful information on how menopausal woman can revive their sex lives, and, funnily, the ones I looked at

---

4 Department of Obstetrics and Gynaecology (2017) '3 tips for better sex after menopause.' Stanford Health, 25 May. Available at: www.stamfordhealth.org/healthflash-blog/womens-health/sex-after-menopause, accessed 17 December 2021.
5 Scott, P. (2016) 'A woman's guide to reviving sex drive.' Available at: www.webmd.com, accessed 17 December 2021.
6 Raypole, C. (2021) 'Yes, you can have an orgasm after menopause – Here's how.' Healthline, 14 May. Available at: www.healthline.com/health/menopause/can-a-woman-have-an-orgasm-after-menopause, accessed 17 December 2021.

all mentioned the use of lubricants and moisturizers as their first point in improving the experience.

At its worse, I had made the choice to abstain from the bedroom gymnastics because I do not believe that 'died during sexual intercourse' should be featured on my death certificate! Now I prepare myself before any sexual encounter, using vaginal moisturizer, rubbing CBD cream on my stiff old hips and dosing myself up with my prescribed painkillers beforehand. It really is such hard work, but I do not consider prepping myself for a fun night with a great partner as a problem. I'm unashamed to say that I am a cougar, and this cougar ain't going down without a fight.

The intention is not to scare anyone into believing that sex is always painful and is practically over once you hit menopause, because some of my friends have told me stories that would make a porn star blush. One girlfriend told me that she traded up for a new sexual partner with more stamina and less attitude and she is having the best sex ever, with no more period interruptions, or children to get in the way. Another said that she no longer has hang-ups about her body, now explores herself intimately and is finally enjoying sex the way she wished she had in her 20s and 30s. I giggled when she said that her husband could no longer keep up with her.

Talking among friends has been so refreshing, enlightening and fun, and should be something we all do because I soon learned that I was not alone in my feelings, worries or tensions.[7] Now I make sure that I speak to both my daughters about the menopause because I want them to be

---

7   Ali, N. (2019) *What We're Told Not to Talk About (But We're Going to Anyway): Women's Voices from East London to Ethiopia.* London: Viking.

prepared and not feel silly, bewildered or confused, and many of the other feelings I experienced from not knowing.

During many of the struggles I have gone through in life, I have always found talking with friends and family a source of comfort, and when it comes to the menopause, it was no different. It is something just about all women, femmes, trans and non-binary people will have to deal with, so bringing it into the open and learning about it is important. I wrongly thought what I considered to be my sexual failures were unique to me, and it was only from speaking with my friends that I realized so many others were affected. Without them, I would never have learned about some of the coping mechanisms and interventions, and that the love him/hate him relationship I had with my partner and my fluctuating libido was a normal part of the menopause journey for so many of us.

16 More to This Than Sweats

Yvonne Christie

I am not sure that I remember a time when my ma didn't sweat or was not sweating. Yet logic tells me there must have been a time. She was 30 years old when I was born, the sixth of her nine birth children, and the last to be born in Jamaica before we moved to the UK in 1955, joining my dad.

As with most youngers I just toodled along, fitting into the order of the times, which was that children should be seen and not heard, especially when visitors came around. My childhood was probably the same as many households – if we were lucky, there was a kitchen, with a conservatory that was added on to the kitchen around the back, which is typical of those times. It was either freezing cold in the winter or steaming hot in the summer months. We had a living room with a TV and a front room, which was for guests, but as we grew and went to secondary and grammar schools, some of us were allowed to study in there.

It is this separation of adults and children that would allow my ma and her sisters and other visiting females who were mainly nurses from the local hospital in East Birmingham where we lived to have private conversations about life. Sometimes it was in whispered tones, but many a time huge laughter would ring out into our ears, and I would wish to join in. Alas, the only time my sister and I could venture into that room when visitors were there was to bring them biscuits and cups of tea in the teapot from the cabinet. As we entered, if there was juicy talk, they would lower their voices until we left the room to join the other siblings who would sometimes want to know 'Who is in there?'

Definitely an air of 'we are the adults, and you are the pleb children, too young to hear the workings of our superior minds' – that's my interpretation of it. But you know what? We accepted that we were not allowed to be party to all the information that adults knew, and that same culture happened across society at large, even in schools.

On reflection, I would have had no chance of hearing about the menopause, sex or menstruating either, not that I am sure they even spoke about these things.

My sister was two years and one day older than me, and it was from her that I learned, via *Lady Chatterley's Lover*, a risqué book for the times, and it was this same sister who told me about my 'monthlies'. My mother's take on it when my sister told her that I was bleeding was to show me where to get the Dr Whites (pads) hidden at the foot of her mahogany wardrobe, every month, and 'make sure your brothers and father don't see them'. She told me to wrap them in newspaper and throw them in the outside bin, and that I must no longer be careless around boys. This was all conveyed surreptitiously in whispered tones. I had no idea what this 'monthlies' business was and what being careless around boys meant when I had six brothers and a live-in dad.

Never fear, my sister was there – thank goodness. She showed me how to properly hook on my Dr Whites with the belt – how cumbersome! After that first showing, my monthlies were very easy to assess, as every month for two to three days my pain would have me groaning and writhing. The plus to this horrendous period happenings was the attention my ma would give me, which is not so easy when you have many other siblings who also warranted her attention. Memories enable me to still relish hot tomato soup and potato mashed with real butter, with the added pleasure of being waited on, so for much of my teen years I felt nurtured and well looked after by my very busy mother.

I lead in with this memory as a way of painting the picture of the improbability of my ma talking about sex and body changes as a female in an open and non-embarrassing way. I just cannot imagine that she would ever be able to have given much thought to the menopause. Might she even have known about it? I mean, she knew about sweating because she had a rag in her petticoat strap, one rag under her pillow, and her handbags always had very nice cotton handkerchiefs, which I'm sure were much too small for the task in hand, but would have been good enough for dabbing her top lip, as ladies of those times often did. Only much later did she have the confidence to have male-sized kerchiefs instead, which were more apt for Sweaty Bettys like my ma and me.

My really painful periods continued right through until my early 20s when I gave birth to my son, but I still would have a bad period here and there, and a blood clot here and there, but mainly I settled down, as do most of us females, to this inconsiderate monthly happening that seemed to be the bane of my life. Because I had an elder, knowledgeable sister with me, I didn't really fear menstruation, unlike my Irish best friend at school, who burst into tears when her periods showed their not-so-pretty face after gym one day. She had no idea what was going on and was so inconsolable that she was allowed to go home early, which was a rarity in those school days. Mind you, those were the days of school nurses and designated sick rooms, where I would often while away an afternoon rubbing my belly and groaning should I have been unfortunate to start bleeding during school hours. The school nurses were always nice and kind, and would give me a blanket so I could drift off to sleep.

Anybody who has ever watched the play or read the book *Vagina Monologues* will understand and acknowledge the number of varying names which we give our vagina. I refer endearingly to mine as my 'min'. I'm not sure where and how the term started, but that is what I have called mine forever and a day. My inners always felt very delicate and my 'min' even more so when the thick and bulky Dr Whites would chafe the hell outta me. Some of this 'min' destruction was also because schools in those days used toilet paper that felt like a baking sheet! Crisp and harsh, causing a rash when used. When I did have a period and went to the school loo, I wasn't cleaning myself like I would do now, with tissue. Cleaning at school meant ripping my very delicate 'min' to shreds, aided and abetted by the nappy-sized Dr Whites that I usually kept on all day as the toilets just did not accommodate themselves to delicate females with body fluids that needed sorting.

I would try really hard to treat my 'min' like the delicate temple that it was, but I suffered with thrush because I actually really adored sex and that would sometimes chafe me. Looking back, I had a pretty average body experience because nothing major interrupted either my libido or disturbed my inners. In my 30s, just before I was sterilized after having my daughter, I donated some eggs because I felt that two children was enough for me as I only had two hands.

As time moved on, I am not sure how I learned about perimenopause and menopause, but I worked in the voluntary sector and often read health articles, women's magazines, and such like. So, when my body started feeling 'weird' and out of synch and I was not sleeping well, as well as my periods messing about left, right and centre – sometimes a yucky beetroot blobby mess, often bleeding for days, and other times just spotting (I can't remember all the details), but I probably was also sweating more around that time – I checked things out with my all-knowing sister who said that her periods were weird too. We spoke about it off and on for a few months and then, feeling fed up with not really knowing what was going on, I had a blood test via my GP to find out if I was dying, or at the very least to find out what was really happening. The GP let me know that I was perimenopausal, and thankfully by then I had already read a book about the menopause, how to go through it naturally, and the importance of diet, rest and exercise. The book had information about the Chinese, Caribbean or West Indian (as many elders used to call it) and other communities across the world whose diets are different to those in the West. Once I knew my weird changes were about the menopause I instantly felt better, and I was mentally equipped to understand that I could just roll with this phase of my life. It's the not knowing what is happening with my body that throws me into panic, with my imagination running wild that it may be cancer and/or death!

When the GP heard that I was also having sleep issues that were probably because I was a working mother of two children, she offered me HRT (hormone replacement therapy), but the only thing I knew about HRT at that time was that I did not want it! There was much in the press at that time about its links to breast cancer. But the real reason I didn't want it is that I am not a great believer in taking pharmaceutical medicine without first trying herbs and alternatives such as exercise or supplements. My mom, being Jamaican, had arrived in the UK with a black mid-sized patent-looking case, and ensconced inside were oils, herbs, rubs for the body and other concoctions that she had brought over with her.

Anything that was wrong with us as children, whether it was worms or liver spots or a cough and a cold, my mom would mix, stir, rub us down or make some special tea to make us better. Those were the days when people coming from the Caribbean could bring in perishables such as herbs and yams, cocoa and ackee in little plastic bags. Back then, it was not considered smuggling! Over the years, my ma did, of course, succumb to the lure of the doctor's surgery, and when she got diabetes, which interestingly developed in the UK, she managed it with shared care using the insulin from the GP and diabetes clinic, backed up by her own herb selection that she got on her visits to pure health shops in London.

My mum lived with diabetes for 50 years and died at 86

– she was a strong old birdie – so my influence in relation to health is not to move to pharmaceutical medicines, and as the menopause seemed to me to be a natural process of womanhood, the HRT journey was not a journey that I was going to travel down easily.

The 'men o pause' – I used to wonder why it is even called that and not 'woman o pause', because I dislike the link to men. The process of female changes has nothing to do with men, and I know that this word was coined by a man and the pause component is because it is often likened to the period of our life when we are no longer necessarily focused on men and them on us, hence the pause. We often see maleness creeping into our lives under the cover of intelligence and academia, but I digress...

I embrace the menopause in my life as a Jamaican who believes in the Universe, coming from a herbal background, and who believes that Black women are glorious with or without interference and should therefore step into whatever phase comes our way. In practice, my naturalness has meant that due to hormone changes I can often have a 'faint' or 'full' moustache, which, with threading and tweezers, is not really a big deal. It is sometimes embarrassing as my 'au naturel' stance means that my top lip can shimmer silver and shiny, so people try to brush dust off my face when what is really needed is a pair of tweezers and for me to put my glasses on so that I can see the hairs and have a yank!

I do not believe that I got moody or more miserable, and if I did, people forgot to tell me, but I'm already quite a straight talker (hopefully not backed up with too much rudeness), although over the years I have had to expand my verbal repertoire so that whoever I am speaking to does not go away with the wrong impression. I often have to remind myself that English is not my first language – it is Jamaican patois – so my dialect can be a bit clumsy, abrupt and less around the corner, which is a very British way to be. So my abruptness is not connected with menopausal mood swings.

The thing that I have noticed more about my experience is that I have a terribly dry 'min', which has cracked and looks scraped, as though someone has taken a small razor blade to it. Looking in the mirror I could see that it got red and bulbous just from walking. One day, my 'min' was so mashed up that I had to hobble into the chemist's and ask for a private room and conversation with the pharmacist so she could supply me with something just to get me home. It was worse than when I had the Dr Whites chafing because it was on the inside of the vagina and not just on the vulva. There are many products for the hormone changes that take place as we mature, and as my 'min' is very delicate, I had to find moisturizer creams with fewer additives or make them myself so that my 'min' could be lubricated. Black women are used to greasing their bodies from top to bottom, but this was about ensuring that I properly moisturize the vulva and vagina. Sometimes I take it for granted that everything is fine and forget to do the routine, only for the dryness to return and I have to start all over again.

Unfortunately, a prolapse has also set in on my 'min'. I discovered that there are many reasons why this can happen, and as I write, I am sitting uncomfortably on a pink lump that likes to protrude through the lips of my 'min'. My pro- lapse has popped back and forth and hasn't really given me much trouble, but I do regret not listening properly to the visiting midwife who used to come to my flat after I had my son and lecture on the importance of pelvic exercises. At the time, being young and arrogant, I didn't feel that I would have a problem with holding my wee or stopping myself in mid flow, which is one of the recommended exercises. As a young person, I felt I knew best so I did not practise regularly, if at all, but I noticed that when doing exercise such as star jumps I would leak a bit of wee. Over the years since then, I have done regular exercises, many of which have included pelvic lifts and holds, but nothing has resolved my current problem of this small apricot-sized prolapse popping out to annoy me whenever it feels like it.

I have been told that I strain to empty my bladder, but do I? This is the main irritant, and I am still unsure how to resolve it as I continue to do pelvic thrusts'n'tilts and I stop my wee in mid flow when I want to, so I guess I must have some pelvic floor muscle.

There is a solution for most things, but I am not going to have an operation that involves netting (plastic netting at that) that some women have resorted to. I know it has caused a large number of middle-aged women big problems as the netting has sometimes fused around feminine organs, leaving women in excruciating pain. My prolapse isn't painful; it is sometimes awkward, and I don't think I'm simplifying it merely because it's a part of my life. I hope that I am speaking my truth and not trying to be a strong Black woman who lives with unnecessary trauma. My reality is that I'm not into pain as I have a low tolerance threshold and I cannot imagine that I would put up with a painful occurrence. I remember how quickly I ducked into the chemist's when my 'min' was being scratched to death, and how I had two to three days off every month because of period pains.

I am not sure what my resolution will be in the long run because it is happening more frequently, but in the short term, how I deal with it is to push the cherry-apricot back up with a clean finger, and from time to time to look at the colour of it in my hand mirror to ensure it's not looking dishevelled or out of sorts. It sounds gross but it is my body, and who better than me to grope and probe using my own hands.

These days I have no sex life, which is mainly through choice – I think! And I sometimes wonder if I would be so generous of mind and self-assessing if I was partaking in regular sex. I'm not sure if it will hurt so I could probably just move over to the side to embrace any sex that ventured my way, but now that the prolapse is more regular, who knows how I would deal with things if sex came my way again.

If you asked me if the menopause was terrifying and scary and took over my life, the answer would be no! It has changed my life and given me freedoms that I never had before, and I save on buying pads and tampons which are very expensive.

Black women have been the bedrock of family life and our wider community, and we will continue to be so, even with the transformations and ageing of our bodies.

Further Reading and Online Resources

ACAS working for everyone: www.acas.org.uk/menopause-at-work

Black Girl Bliss (2018) *Pussy Prayers: Sacred and Sensual Rituals for Wild Women of Colour*. Independently published.

Black Girl's Guide to Surviving Menopause: https://blackgirl sguidetosurvivingmenopause.com

Black Menopause and Beyond: www.instagram.com/ blkmenobeyond

Black Menopause and Beyond podcast with Anita Powell: https://shows.acast.com/black-menopause-and-beyond

Black Women in Health UK: www.bwih.co.uk/blog

Black Women in Menopause founded by Nina Kuypers: www.blackhealthandbeyond.co.uk/copy-of-black-women-in-menopause

Black Women's Health Imperative USA: https://bwhi.org/ videos

Brewer, S., Jones, M.L. and Eichenwald, T. (2007) *Menopause for Dummies*. Chichester: John Wiley & Sons Ltd.

British Menopause Society (2022) Menopause Practice Standards. Available at https://thebms.org.uk/wp-content/ uploads/2022/12/BMS-Menopause-Practice-Standards-DEC2022-A.pdf, accessed 24 January 2023.

CIPD Menopause at Work: www.cipd.co.uk/knowledge/ culture/well-being/menopause/printable-resources

Destigmatising Black Menopause Experiences: www. youandmenopause.org/blog

Eltahawy, M. (2021) 'Menopause chicks.' Feminist Giant, 7 December. Available at www.feministgiant.com/p/--7ed, accessed 31 August 2022.

Hot Flash (2012) 'Nutrition for menopause.' Podcast. Available at: www.scribd.com/podcast/418050243/Hot-Flash-Nutrition-for-Menopause-This-week-Dar-Kvist-and-Kara-Carper-discuss-ways-to-prevent-the-unpleasant-symptoms-that-menopause-can-bring-about, accessed 31 August 2022.

International Menopause Society: www.imsociety.org/for-women

Leonard, R. (2017) *Menopause – The Answers: Understand and Manage Symptoms with Natural Solutions, Alternative Remedies and Conventional Medical Advice*. London: Orion Spring.

Lewis, J. (2018) *Me and My Menopausal Vagina*. PAL Books.

MAMM (Maureen Anderson Menopause Moments): www.maureen-anderson.co.uk/what-i-do/mamm-menopause-moments

Menopause NHS Choices: www.nhs.uk/Conditions/Menopause/Pages/Introduction.aspx

Menopause Whilst Black podcast with Karen Arthur: https://podcasts.apple.com/gb/podcast/menopause-whilst-black/id1537012198

Muir, K. (2022) *Everything you need to know about the menopause (but were too afraid to ask)*. London: Gallery UK.

Muneeza: https://muneezaahmed.com/the-mysteries-of-menstruation-menopause-why-all-the-drama

Peppy Health: https://info.peppyhealth.com/peppy-menopause-resources

Queer Menopause: www.queermenopause.com/resources

Raymond-Williams, R. (2021) *More Than Talk: Perspectives of Black and People of Colour Working in Sexual and Reproductive Health in the United Kingdom*. Independently published.

Rock My Menopause: https://rockmymenopause.com/get-informed/transgender-health

Scott Brown, C. and Levy, B. (2004) *The Black Woman's Guide to Menopause: Doing Menopause with Heart and Soul*. Naperville, IL: Sourcebooks, Inc.

The Daisy Network: www.daisynetwork.org

The Society of Obstetricians and Gynaecologists of Canada (SOGC): www.menopauseandu.ca

Troughton, M. (2007) *Magical Menopause: 52 Brilliant Ideas for Celebrating Your New Life*. Oxford: The Infinite Ideas Company Limited.

Contributor Biographies

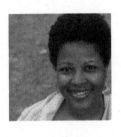

Iya Rev. DeShannon Barnes-Bowens, M.S.

I am the founder of ILERA Counseling & Education Services, where I work as a psychotherapist, professional development trainer and spiritual counsellor. I offer workshops and programmes focusing on sexuality and spirituality, sexual abuse and healing, and vicarious trauma and wellness. I am the author of *Hush Hush: An African American Family Breaks their Silence on Sexuality and Sexual Abuse* (2007, 2015), and an ordained Interfaith minister. I am also an initiated priestess in the Ifa-Orisa spiritual tradition and enjoy guiding others in their journey of freedom. To find out more, visit http://ilera.com

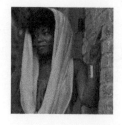

Onika Henry

I am a trained educator, facilitator, coun-sellor and theatre artist with university qualifications in Theatre Arts, Psych-ology and Human Sexuality, and I live on the island Tobago (of Trinidad and Tobago in the Caribbean). I was a 2019 TEDx Port of Spain Speaker, a USA Fulbright Scholar (2012) and I am the co-founder of a top perform-ing arts company in Tobago. I am a contributing writer for the *Tobago Newsday* newspaper, and volunteer at a few non-governmental organizations, including Tobago's only halfway home for ex-prisoners and deportees. As a strong proponent of Theatre for Development (TfD) and Applied Arts, I actively use the arts as a tool for social and behaviour change.

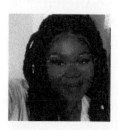

Shaneka Lambert

I am a 27-year-old Black woman. I am currently a support worker and foster carer based in England. I have a passion for exercise and supporting young people transitioning into adulthood. I have big dreams and ambitions for myself, and I am currently working towards owning my own business in the near future. I intend to support others who, like me, have experienced early meno-pause, and I am planning to explore different routes to help me with my fertility treatment.

Nicole Joseph-Chin

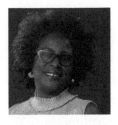

I am a breast care specialist, social impact strategist and health justice advocate with over two decades of experience in breast advocacy, towards catalysing global social change in women's health, reproductive health and gender justice. As CEO of Ms Brafit Limited I find solutions for women, girls, medical practitioners and women in treatment, and offer educational programming on bra fittings, breast care consultations, post-surgical bra fittings (mastectomy, elective surgeries, lumpectomies or investigative surgical procedures), retail solutions, educational programming (corporate, industry, grassroots and schools), professional consultancy and policy development and design.

Palmela Witter

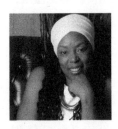

My name is Palmela. I am not a Pamela! I am a first-generation British-born Sister and the eldest of five siblings whose parents migrated from British Guiana (now called Guyana). I am a proud mother to three adult children (one son and twin daughters), and a grandmother. The grandsons are the light of my life, and it is their zest for life that has encouraged me to continue my international travelling by setting the task that we journey to as many Caribbean countries and islands as possible. I love cooking a good pot of Guyanese curry and, dare I say it, am still learning to 'clap' the roti, but my grandsons are getting the hang of it. I am now inspired to continue my academic studies and pursue my story writing.

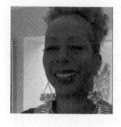

Yansie Rolston

I am a mental health and wellbeing advocate and practitioner with a depth of experience and expertise in health equality and service development. To further my knowledge about the diversity and intersectionality of menopause, I have travelled to the USA, South America, the Caribbean and Africa, listening to the stories, immersing myself in the experiences of local people and engaging with healthcare practitioners. I am a member of the British Menopause Society. As a Heyoka empath, my intuition and sensitivity are heightened so I often go against convention, questioning and challenging societal norms, and spending time championing social justice. I love reading a good biography – the ones that you don't want to put down even when your bladder is full to capacity and your brain is saying 'open sesame'.

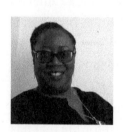

Yvonne Witter

I love and appreciate enabling clients to unravel their confusion around policy and practice by assisting them to fulfil their dreams as business owners. I have enabled thousands of new starts and capacity-built many organizations working within the private and social enterprise sectors and across geographical boundaries. I enable organizations that are stuck in their processes to achieve clarity around what is possible, by devising tools to use in ensuring objectives are met. I would describe myself as a conscious practitioner seeking client satisfaction. I am a published author, and write both fiction and non-fiction. I love travelling, creative arts, writing, food and good conversation. My most recent publication, *Developing Customer Service in the Black Owned Business*, is available online.

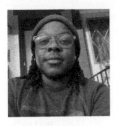

Austen Smith

I am a masculine-of-centre, non-binary storyteller, qualitative researcher and radical imagination doula. My work explores the philosophical elements of dreamwork, menopause, Black gender proliferation, post-activism and ancestral veneration as freedom practices born of the technologies of Blackness. Growing up, I always thought rituals were performed either in the church or in secret. The mysterious air around ritualism made it feel holy beyond measure, too pure for a common consumer like myself. No one told me ritual would be the bridge that could connect me to my ancestors, my culture, my community, myself.

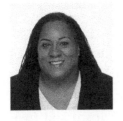

Jacqueline Hinds

I am the founder of the Society of Emotional Intelligence International UK & Europe and a Certified Emotional Intelligence coach, who is passionate about people – supporting their emotional health and wellbeing needs by providing coaching, training and developmental initiatives to help them to realize, unlock and release their true potential to be the best they can be. I believe that there is a significant paradigm shift across the mental health and wellbeing arena, and that self-care is essential and necessary right now. My hope and prayer by sharing my lived experience and that of others through my writing is that it will be of comfort and support to others.

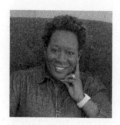

Sandra Wilson

I am a wife and mother and a keen advocate of whole life living, with a large dose of laughter, fun and enjoyment-in-the-moment experiences. I am an accredited senior practitioner coach and coach supervisor, and support organizations and the wider community to raise awareness of menopause, helping them in developing workplace policies that support the workforce. I am passionate about empowering others to develop individual strategies to fulfil their personal wellbeing goals that are integral to all that they do.

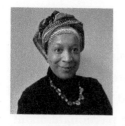

Mbeke Waseme

I am an international author, photographer, coach and freelance writer, and my publications include *How to Live, Work and Thrive Abroad* (2022) and two poetry books, *Exploring All of Me* (2019) and *And Then It Was 2020* (2020). I have contributed chapters, poems, essays and academic articles in a number of publications. My articles and photographs have been featured in the *African Business and Culture Magazine* (now called *Nex Generation*), *The Alarm Magazine*, *Diversity Business Promotes*, *Turning Points* magazine, and Black Ballad, and in 2020, I released recorded poems. I have lived and worked in Ghana, strengthening and growing teacher and leadership capacity through coaching, mentoring, training and facilitating action learning sets.

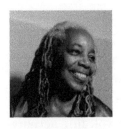

Asma-Esmeralda Abdallah-Portales

I am a Black, queer, transcultural activist. A native Cuban, I arrived in Germany with my parents at the age of six. Among other things, I have worked as a translator and cultural mediator. Most recently, I have worked as a counsellor at the refugee office of Kargah eV. I was also actively involved in the Initiative of Black People in Germany (ISD), but have since has moved back to Cuba where I am active in feminist circles and provide support to Afro-Cuban activists and the LGBTIQ community. My areas of study are psychology, feminist literary theory and gender studies and Cuban studies.

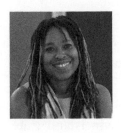

Pamela Windle

I have a BSc in Psychology and Sport Science, and I am an integrated certified international women's health coach, speaker and menopause in the workplace consultant, with 20+ years of experience in the health and wellness sector. I have trained with the Integrated Women's Health Institute and the International Menopause Society, and I am a member of the British Standard Institute and co-creator of a menstruation to menopause policy in the workplace. My passion is supporting and empowering women in perimenopause, menopause and beyond, and I use evidence-based practice to combine training and techniques with organizations, individual needs and senior leaders.

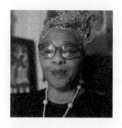

Myrle Roach

Born on the Caribbean island of Montserrat, with a passion for theatre, drama and creative writing, I migrated to the UK in 2002 following volcanic activity on the island. I then began to focus more on creative writing and have had poems published in an anthology, *Brown Eyes*, along with articles in regional publications. In 2018 I published my first book of poetry, *Tamarind Seeds*, and have been performing poetry in the Midlands and London under the stage name of 'Alliouagana Pearl', Alliouagana being the Amerindian Arawak name for Montserrat. You can check out my website at www.alliouaganapearl.com and follow me on social media.

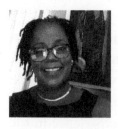

Leslie Anne Bishop, MBBS, DA (UWI), DPH (Liverpool), FRCOG

I am an African-Caribbean woman currently living on the twin island state of Trinidad and Tobago, 10 years postmenopause and a practising gynaecologist in the Caribbean since 1996. My undergraduate training was at the Faculty of Medicine, University of the West Indies, and my post-graduate gynaecology training was in the UK. Knowledge is power. Educating ourselves about our health is essential to achieving our right to 'complete physical, mental and social well-being'.[1]

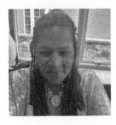

Tashini Jones

My friends would hopefully describe me as loyal and honest; my kids would describe me as cantankerous; and I would definitely say I am truthful and just tell it how it is. My health challenges and other life events have made me alter the way that I used to handle situations and now I no longer sugar-coat things. I say it as I see it without intent to cause offence. I come from a training and development background, and spent my working career imparting information and sharing knowledge. My interests are human nutrition, biomedical sciences and music.

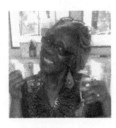

Yvonne Christie

I identify as a Jamaican-Brummie and I love the feeling of saying that I am retired after 40+ years as a community development worker advocating for

1   WHO (World Health Organization) (1946) 'Constitution of the World Health Organization.' *American Journal of Public Health and Nations Health 36*, 1315–1323. https://doi.org/10.2105/AJPH.36.11.1315

change in Black mental health as a practitioner and as a critical spokeswoman. I recognize that there are many development areas that keep us mentally strong and feed our wellbeing, so these days I'm happy walking my two dogs on the coast of Kent, taking on a slowed-down pace of life, which I'm gradually beginning to recognize that I deserve, although I still try my hand at creative opportunities that come my way!